Autism Diagnosis
An Artificial Intelligence Approach

AF839591

Editors:
Wellington Pinheiro dos Santos
Associate Professor, Department of Biomedical Engineering
Universidade Federal de Pernambuco, Brazil

Flávio Secco Fonseca
Doctoral Researcher, Polytechnic School of Pernambuco
Universidade de Pernambuco, Brazil

Juliana Carneiro Gomes
Associate Professor, Department of Biomedical Engineering
Universidade Federal de Pernambuco, Brazil

Maíra Araújo de Santana
Associate Professor, Department of Biomedical Engineering
Universidade Federal de Pernambuco, Brazil

CRC Press
Taylor & Francis Group
Boca Raton London New York

CRC Press is an imprint of the
Taylor & Francis Group, an **informa** business
A SCIENCE PUBLISHERS BOOK

First edition published 2026
by CRC Press
2385 NW Executive Center Drive, Suite 320, Boca Raton FL 33431

and by CRC Press
4 Park Square, Milton Park, Abingdon, Oxon, OX14 4RN

CRC Press is an imprint of Taylor & Francis Group, LLC

Library of Congress Cataloging-in-Publication Data (applied for)

ISBN: 978-1-032-85120-4 (hbk)
ISBN: 978-1-032-87208-7 (pbk)
ISBN: 978-1-003-53141-8 (ebk)

DOI: 10.1201/9781003531418

Typeset in Times New Roman
by Prime Publishing Services

Preface
Toward a Multidisciplinary Future in Autism Detection and Support

"I slept and dreamt that life was joy. I awoke and saw that life was service. I acted and behold, service was joy."

—Rabindranath Tagore

Autism Spectrum Disorder (ASD) is one of the most complex and prevalent neurodevelopmental conditions affecting individuals across the globe. With an estimated prevalence of 1 in 100 children worldwide, ASD encompasses a wide range of manifestations, including differences in social interaction, communication, sensory processing, and behavioral patterns. These characteristics are present from early childhood and vary significantly among individuals, making each case unique and requiring tailored approaches to diagnosis, support, and intervention.

In recent decades, the scientific and clinical communities have made significant strides in understanding ASD. However, challenges remain—particularly in ensuring timely detection and providing equitable access to diagnostic tools and therapeutic interventions. Early identification remains a critical factor in enabling effective, individualized support that can significantly improve developmental outcomes and quality of life for individuals on the spectrum and their families.

This evolving landscape has been increasingly shaped by technological advancements and interdisciplinary collaboration. Artificial Intelligence (AI), biomedical engineering, applied neuroscience, and clinical practice are converging to develop more accurate, accessible, and personalized solutions for autism detection and care. These innovations not only enhance diagnostic precision but also open new pathways for understanding brain function, behavior, and human development.

The integration of these disciplines reflects a broader shift toward holistic, inclusive, and ethically grounded approaches to neurodiversity—one where technology serves as a tool for empowerment rather than normalization, and where early detection becomes a gateway to meaningful, lifelong support.

Purpose and Scope of the Book

This edited volume was conceived with a clear mission: to bridge existing knowledge gaps in ASD detection and intervention by fostering interdisciplinary dialogue and innovation. The complexity of ASD demands a holistic approach—one that transcends traditional disciplinary boundaries and integrates insights from clinical neuroscience, biomedical engineering, AI, and human-centered developmental models.

Over the years, significant progress has been made in understanding the neurobiological and behavioral aspects of autism. However, many challenges persist, particularly in ensuring early, accurate, and accessible diagnosis across diverse populations. Technological advancements offer promising solutions, yet their integration into real-world clinical and educational settings remains fragmented. This book seeks to address these challenges by offering a unified perspective that brings together foundational knowledge, cutting-edge methodologies, and ethical considerations.

The chapters in this volume reflect a carefully curated journey through the evolving landscape of autism research and practice. Beginning with historical and clinical foundations, it moves through current diagnostic frameworks and explores how emerging technologies—such as EEG-based signal processing, machine learning, deep learning, and Explainable AI—are reshaping detection paradigms. The book also delves into innovative tools like wearables, virtual reality, and intelligent platforms that support both clinicians and families.

Crucially, the volume does not stop at technological innovation. It emphasizes the importance of humanistic and developmental approaches, such as the DIR/Floortime model, which prioritize individuality, emotional engagement, and relational growth. By integrating these perspectives, the book advocates for systems that do not merely detect autism but understand and support the unique ways in which individuals on the spectrum experience and interact with the world.

In doing so, this work aims to inspire researchers, practitioners, and policymakers to adopt a more inclusive, multidisciplinary, and ethically grounded vision of autism care—one where technology serves as a tool for empowerment rather than normalization, and where early detection becomes a gateway to lifelong, person-centered support.

Overview of Content Organization

The structure of this book reflects a carefully curated progression from foundational knowledge to cutting-edge innovations in ASD detection and support. Each chapter contributes a distinct yet complementary perspective, building a comprehensive and multidisciplinary understanding of autism research, diagnosis, and intervention.

Chapter 1 provides a brief overview of key concepts AI, machine learning, and applied neuroscience. Chapters 2 and 3 lay the essential groundwork by offering a historical and clinical overview of ASD, tracing its evolving conceptualization from early descriptions by Kanner and Asperger to modern diagnostic criteria. These chapters examine global prevalence rates, gender disparities, and sociocultural barriers that influence access to timely diagnosis. They also underscore the critical importance of early detection and intervention in improving long-term outcomes for individuals on the spectrum.

Chapter 4 shifts the focus toward human-centered therapeutic approaches, introducing the DIR/Floortime model as a relational, developmentally sensitive framework. It challenges behaviorist paradigms that prioritize normalization over individuality and advocates for practices that honor emotional engagement, autonomy, and developmental uniqueness.

Chapters 5 through 7 delve into the technological frontier of ASD detection. These chapters explore how biomedical signal processing—particularly using electroencephalography (EEG)—can be combined with machine learning and deep learning techniques to identify neurophysiological patterns associated with autism. Chapter 5 provides a narrative review of AI-based strategies applied to EEG data, while Chapter 6 presents an innovative methodology that integrates wavelet transforms with hybrid deep learning models for improved classification accuracy. Chapter 7 addresses practical implementation challenges by proposing optimized, low-density EEG configurations using feature selection and interpolation techniques, making advanced diagnostics more accessible in real-world settings.

Chapter 8 expands the technological scope by reviewing emerging innovations such as wearable devices, virtual and augmented reality, Internet of Things (IoT), and ontology-based modeling. The chapter emphasizes the role of Explainable Artificial Intelligence (XAI) in ensuring transparency and interpretability in AI-assisted decision-making, aligning technical advancements with ethical and clinical needs.

Finally, Chapter 9 offers a philosophical and ethical reflection on the integration of artificial intelligence in autism care. Drawing from personal narratives and theoretical frameworks, it explores how AI systems—especially large language models—can serve as interactive partners rather than mere diagnostic tools. It calls for ethically grounded, neurodiversity-affirming technologies that enhance relational ethics and promote dignity, inclusion, and personalized support.

Together, these chapters form a cohesive narrative that bridges science and humanity, technology and empathy, diagnosis and development. This multidisciplinary journey reflects our shared commitment to advancing autism detection and support through innovation, inclusivity, and integrity.

Target Audience

This book is designed to serve a broad and diverse audience, reflecting the inherently multidisciplinary nature of ASD detection and support. It will be of particular interest to researchers in neuroscience, biomedical engineering, AI, and developmental psychology, who are actively engaged in advancing diagnostic methodologies and therapeutic tools.

Clinicians and healthcare professionals, including pediatricians, psychiatrists, neuropsychologists, and speech-language pathologists, will find valuable insights into emerging technologies that can enhance early diagnosis and improve clinical decision-making. The integration of AI-based tools with traditional assessment methods offers practical applications for everyday practice, especially in resource-constrained environments.

For educators, special education professionals, and school psychologists, the volume provides essential knowledge on how technological advancements—such as intelligent tutoring systems, wearable devices, and virtual reality—can be leveraged to create inclusive learning environments and support neurodivergent students more effectively.

The content is also highly relevant to engineers and AI developers working at the intersection of machine learning, signal processing, and healthcare. Chapters detailing EEG-based classification models, deep learning architectures, and explainable AI strategies offer technical depth while addressing real-world implementation challenges such as data scarcity, model interpretability, and ethical deployment.

Policymakers and public health officials will benefit from discussions around equitable access to diagnostic tools, the role of technology in reducing disparities, and the importance of integrating scientific innovation with social inclusion policies.

Finally, this book serves as a comprehensive reference for graduate students and early-career researchers across multiple disciplines, offering both foundational knowledge and cutting-edge developments in autism research and detection.

By bridging theory and practice, science and ethics, this volume aims to empower professionals across academic, clinical, educational, and technological domains, fostering a shared commitment to advancing ASD detection through interdisciplinary collaboration and human-centered innovation.

Editorial Vision and Motivation

As editors, our motivation for compiling this volume stems from a shared vision: to bridge the worlds of science and humanity, to foster inclusive innovation, and to promote accessible, equitable care for individuals across the autism spectrum. ASD is not only a subject of scientific inquiry but also a deeply human experience—one that calls for empathy, ethical responsibility, and a commitment to understanding each individual's unique way of being in the world.

This book emerged from a recognition that while technological advancements are accelerating at an unprecedented pace, their true value lies not in the sophistication of algorithms or the precision of diagnostic tools, but in how they serve people, particularly those who have historically been underserved or misunderstood. We believe that progress must be measured not only by accuracy rates or computational efficiency but also by inclusion, dignity, and ethical engagement.

One of the central motivations behind this work has been to challenge the notion that autism must be "detected to correct". Instead, we advocate for a paradigm where detection becomes a pathway to understanding, support, and empowerment. This requires moving beyond standardized behavioral models and embracing approaches that respect neurodiversity, celebrate individual strengths, and prioritize relational development—such as the DIR/Floortime model explored in Chapter 3.

We are also deeply aware of the cultural, economic, and social disparities that shape access to diagnosis and intervention. In many regions, families face long waiting times, lack of trained professionals, and limited resources—barriers that technology can help overcome if designed with equity in mind. Chapters such as 6 and 8 highlight the importance of adapting AI and biomedical tools to real-world conditions, ensuring that innovations do not widen existing gaps but instead contribute to more democratic and inclusive healthcare systems.

Responsible innovation, therefore, is not just a technical challenge: it is an ethical imperative. It demands transparency in AI, sensitivity in data interpretation, and cultural humility in clinical application. As reflected in Chapter 8, we see AI not as a replacement for human connection but as a potential ally in expanding access to meaningful support. When guided by principles of relational ethics and neurodiversity-affirming practices, technology can become a tool for empowerment rather than normalization.

Ultimately, this book represents a call for integration—not only across disciplines, but also across values. It invites researchers, clinicians, educators, engineers, and policymakers to collaborate in ways that honor both scientific rigor and human dignity. Our hope is that this volume will inspire future work that continues to push the boundaries of what is possible, always grounded in the belief that every individual deserves to be seen, understood, and supported on their own terms.

Key Contributions and Innovations

This book presents a rich tapestry of innovations that collectively advance the field of ASD detection, diagnosis, and support. Each chapter contributes distinct methodological, technological, and philosophical insights, while also reinforcing shared themes that point to the future of multidisciplinary autism research.

One of the most notable technical contributions comes from Chapters 5 through 7, which explore cutting-edge approaches to EEG-based ASD classification. These chapters demonstrate how wavelet transforms can be used to convert complex EEG signals into image-like representations suitable for deep learning analysis. Chapter 6, in particular, introduces a hybrid architecture combining Convolutional Neural Networks (CNNs) such as GoogLeNet and VGG16 with Bidirectional Gated Recurrent Units (BiGRUs), offering a novel pipeline for identifying neurophysiological patterns associated with autism. Although early results show room for improvement in accuracy, the model demonstrates high sensitivity, suggesting its potential as a complementary diagnostic tool.

A major step toward real-world applicability appears in Chapter 7, where the authors tackle the challenge of reducing the number of EEG channels required for accurate classification. By employing feature selection techniques like Particle Swarm Optimization (PSO) and handling missing data through Inverse Distance Weighting (IDW), they propose a streamlined, low-density EEG configuration that retains diagnostic performance. This innovation opens the door to more accessible, cost-effective, and portable tools for ASD screening—especially in resource-limited environments.

Beyond the realm of signal processing and machine learning, Chapter 4 brings an essential human-centered perspective to the conversation. It introduces the DIR/Floortime model, emphasizing emotional engagement, relational development, and individualized therapeutic pathways. This chapter serves as a vital counterpoint to purely algorithmic approaches, reminding us that technology should not only detect but also understand and support the unique ways in which individuals with ASD experience the world.

Looking ahead to next-generation technologies, Chapter 8 explores the integration of XAI, Retrieval-Augmented Generation (RAG), and Large Language Models (LLMs) in autism care. These systems hold promise not just for automating diagnosis, but for enhancing communication between clinicians, families, and autistic individuals themselves. The chapter envisions AI-driven chatbots that assist in interpreting behavioral assessments, adapting educational strategies, and supporting clinical decision-making, all while maintaining transparency and interpretability.

Finally, Chapter 9 offers a profound ethical reflection on the role of AI in autism support. Drawing from personal narratives and philosophical frameworks, it argues for neurodiversity-affirming AI that amplifies relational ethics rather than imposing normative standards. The chapter calls for systems that do not define autism but engage with it dialogically, co-creating new ecologies of care that respect difference, foster autonomy, and uphold dignity.

Together, these contributions illustrate the transformative potential of integrating AI, biomedical engineering, applied neuroscience, and developmental psychology. They represent not only technical milestones but also ethical imperatives: to build systems that are inclusive, equitable, and deeply human.

Future Directions

The research and insights presented in this volume not only reflect the current state of ASD detection but also illuminate a promising path forward—one defined by multimodal data fusion, personalized diagnostics, real-time monitoring, and inclusive AI design.

One of the most compelling directions for future research lies in the integration of multimodal data sources—such as EEG, eye-tracking, behavioral markers, genetic profiles, and environmental sensors—to build more comprehensive and accurate models of ASD. As highlighted in Chapters 5 through 7, combining diverse datasets enhances diagnostic sensitivity and reduces reliance on any single modality. The next generation of tools must evolve to handle such complexity while maintaining interpretability and clinical relevance.

Personalization will be key to ensuring that early detection translates into meaningful support. While machine learning and deep learning models have shown promise in identifying general patterns associated with ASD, future systems must adapt to the unique neurophysiological and behavioral signatures of each individual. This shift toward individualized diagnostics aligns with the human-centered developmental models discussed in Chapter 4, particularly the DIR/Floortime framework, which emphasizes relational growth and tailored intervention strategies.

Real-time monitoring, enabled by wearable devices and IoT -based systems, offers another transformative opportunity. As explored in Chapter 8, continuous physiological and behavioral tracking can provide valuable insights into sensory responses, emotional regulation, and developmental trajectories. These technologies pave the way for dynamic, context-aware support systems that go beyond static diagnostic labels to offer adaptive assistance in everyday life.

Crucially, the field must prioritize inclusive AI design—systems that are not only technically robust but also ethically grounded, culturally sensitive, and accessible across diverse populations. Chapter 8 underscores the importance of developing AI that respects neurodiversity rather than imposing normative standards. Future AI applications should function as collaborative partners, supporting clinicians, educators, and families without replacing the relational and contextual dimensions of care.

To realize these advancements, we call for increased interdisciplinary collaboration and translational research that bridges laboratory discoveries with real-world implementation. Researchers in AI, biomedical engineering, neuroscience, and clinical practice must work together with educators, policymakers, and members of the autistic community to ensure that innovations serve genuine needs and promote equity.

As we move forward, our collective goal should be clear: to build a future where autism detection is not only earlier and more accurate but also more humane, inclusive, and empowering for all individuals on the spectrum.

Acknowledgments

This book would not have been possible without the invaluable contributions and support of numerous individuals and institutions. We extend our deepest gratitude to all the chapter authors for their expertise, dedication, and thoughtful insights that brought this multidisciplinary volume to life.

We also acknowledge the generous support of several Brazilian funding agencies, including the National Council for Scientific and Technological Development (CNPq), the Pernambuco State Science and Technology Support Foundation (FACEPE), and the Studies and Projects Financing Agency (FINEP). Their financial assistance has been instrumental in enabling the research and collaborative efforts reflected in this work.

Our sincere appreciation goes to the academic and research institutions that provided the infrastructure and environment necessary for the development of the studies included in this book. We are especially grateful to the reviewers whose constructive feedback significantly strengthened the quality and coherence of the final chapters.

Finally, we wish to express our heartfelt gratitude to the families and individuals living with ASD, who continue to inspire and guide our work. Their resilience, courage, and unique perspectives remind us daily of the profound human impact behind every scientific endeavor. It is for them—and with them—that we strive toward more inclusive, compassionate, and equitable advancements in autism detection and care.

Closing Statement

The journey through this book underscores a powerful truth: the future of ASD detection and support lies in the integration of diverse disciplines—from neuroscience and biomedical engineering to artificial intelligence, developmental psychology, and ethics. By bringing together these fields, we open new pathways not only for earlier and more accurate diagnosis but also for more inclusive, personalized, and compassionate care.

Each chapter contributes to a growing body of knowledge that challenges traditional paradigms and redefines what it means to detect, understand, and support individuals on the autism spectrum. The innovations presented—from advanced EEG signal processing and machine learning models to human-centered therapeutic frameworks and ethically grounded AI—reflect a shared commitment to progress that honors both scientific rigor and human dignity.

As we look ahead, we are filled with hope for a future where technology does not merely categorize or diagnose, but actively supports neurodiversity and empowers individuals to thrive. We envision inclusive healthcare systems that embrace technological advancements while remaining rooted in equity, accessibility, and respect for individual differences. We see a world where early detection becomes a gateway to meaningful intervention, where AI acts as a partner rather than a replacement for human connection, and where every person—regardless of neurotype—is valued and supported.

This volume is not just a collection of research; it is a call to action. A call to researchers to continue pushing boundaries responsibly. A call to clinicians and educators to adopt tools that enhance understanding and inclusion. And a call to society at large to recognize and celebrate neurodiversity as an essential part of our shared human experience.

Together, through collaboration, empathy, and innovation, we can build a future where autism is not only better understood—but also better supported, more inclusively integrated, and deeply respected.

Recife, Brazil, May 30, 2025

Wellington Pinheiro dos Santos,
Flávio Secco Fonseca,
Juliana Carneiro Gomes,
and **Maíra Araújo de Santana**

Contents

List of Contributors

Adrielly Sayonara
Universidade Federal de Pernambuco, Recife, Brazil.

Adrielly Sayonara de Oliveira Silva
Universidade Federal de Pernambuco, Recife, Brazil.

Arthur Moreira Nogueira de Melo
Universidade Federal de Pernambuco, Brazil.

Camila Narjara
Universidade Federal de Pernambuco, Recife, Brazil.

Camila Tiodista de Lima
Universidade Federal de Pernambuco, Recife, Brazil.

Camila Xavier de Medeiros
Universidade Federal de Pernambuco, Brazil.

Carlo Marcelo Revoredo da Silva
Universidade de Pernambuco, Pernambuco, Brazil.

Carol Mota
PhD in Cognitive Psychology, Master's in Education, Cultures, and Identities; DIR/Floortime Therapist.

Desirée Louise Procópio Alves
Neuropediatrician, Brazil

Fabiano Tonaco Borges
Universidade Federal de Pernambuco, Brazil.

Flávio Secco Fonseca
Universidade de Pernambuco, Brazil.

Gabriel Miranda de Souza
Universidade Federal de Pernambuco, Recife, Brazil.

Ingrid Bruno Nunes
Universidade Federal de Pernambuco, Recife, Brazil.

Jordana Leandro Seixas
Universidade de Pernambuco, Brazil.

Júlia Vitória Torres D'Arruda
Universidade Federal de Pernambuco, Recife, Brazil.

Juliana C. Gomes Cassemiro
Universidade Federal de Pernambuco, Recife, Brazil.

Karla Amorim Sancho
Universidade Federal de Pernambuco, Brazil.

Maíra Araújo de Santana
Universidade Federal de Pernambuco, Brazil.

Maria Euclécia Albuquerque da Silva
Universidade Federal de Pernambuco, Recife, Brazil.

Marina Assis Pinheiro
PhD in Psychology, Department of Psychology, Professor at the Federal University of Pernambuco.

Thailson Caetano Valdeci da Silva
Universidade Federal de Pernambuco, Recife, Brazil.

Vanderlene Covre Rocha
Universidade de Pernambuco, Pernambuco, Brazil. or Instituto Federal do Pará, Pará, Brazil.

Wellington Pinheiro dos Santos
Universidade Federal de Pernambuco, Recife, Brazil

Wesley Gregório Machado
Universidade Federal de Pernambuco, Brazil.

1 Introductory Concepts of Neuroscience and Computational Intelligence

Adrielly Sayonara de Oliveira Silva[1*], Gabriel Miranda de Souza[1], Ingrid Bruno Nunes[1], Camila Tiodista de Lima[1], Júlia Vitória Torres D'Arruda[1], Juliana C. Gomes Cassemiro[1], Maíra Araújo de Santana[1] and Wellington Pinheiro dos Santos[1]

This chapter explores the interface between neuroscience and computational intelligence in the investigation of brain function and the development of advanced neurotechnologies. It proposes a comprehensive conceptual framework that integrates biological principles with methodologies derived from artificial intelligence, structured around three core aspects: (1) the neurofunctional bases of brain organization, with an emphasis on distributed processing and network dynamics; (2) electroencephalography (EEG) as a fundamental and accessible method for capturing neural activity with high temporal resolution; and (3) computational intelligence techniques, particularly artificial neural networks and deep learning architectures, employed in the analysis of complex neurophysiological data. The chapter underscores how computational models both influence and are shaped by neuroscientific findings, fostering a reciprocal and cumulative process of knowledge production. Moreover, it presents a detailed examination of the technical characteristics and applications of EEG, followed by a critical analysis of machine learning approaches used for pattern recognition in neural data. The discussion demonstrates how this interdisciplinary convergence eases the emergence of innovative methodologies in brain research, while simultaneously introducing challenges related to model interpretability and alignment with biological principles. Emerging trends and prospective directions are also addressed, including multimodal data integration, the role of explainable artificial intelligence in neuroscience, and the pursuit of more biologically plausible neural models. Our goal is to equip readers with both foundational knowledge and contemporary insights into this dynamic and evolving intersection between brain science and artificial intelligence,

1 Federal University of Pernambuco, Recife, Brazil.
* Corresponding author: adrielly.sayonara@ufpe.br

DOI: 10.1201/9781003531418-1

in which the mutual advancement of both domains continues to redefine the boundaries of inquiry.

1. Introduction

The human brain represents one of the most complex and enigmatic systems in nature, characterized by a highly interconnected neuronal architecture composed of approximately 86 billion neurons that communicate through chemical and electrical synapses (Luo, 2021). This vast and dynamic network gives rise to high-order phenomena such as perception, cognition, behavior, language, emotions, and consciousness. The intrinsic nonlinearity, adaptability, and multiscale organization of neural processes make the comprehensive understanding of brain function a formidable scientific challenge. Traditional reductionist approaches, although valuable, often fall short in capturing the emergent properties of neural systems.

In recent decades, however, the convergence of advances in neuroscience and computational intelligence has profoundly transformed our ability to investigate the human brain (Domenico, 2017). Techniques such as artificial neural networks, deep learning architectures, graph-theoretical modeling, and large-scale data analysis have enabled the development of computational frameworks capable of simulating and interpreting brain activity with unprecedented resolution and complexity (Amunts et al., 2022). These tools allow for the modeling of brain dynamics across multiple spatial and temporal scales, from microcircuits to large-scale functional networks, revealing patterns that are often inaccessible through traditional experimental methods.

This interdisciplinary integration has opened new perspectives for elucidating the mechanisms underlying cognitive functions and neurodevelopmental trajectories. Moreover, it has catalyzed progress in critical domains such as the early diagnosis of neuropsychiatric and neurodevelopmental disorders, including autism spectrum disorder (ASD) and Alzheimer's disease, personalized cognitive rehabilitation, and the refinement of neurotechnologies, particularly brain–machine interfaces (BMIs). The use of data-driven approaches and biologically inspired models not only enhances the explanatory power of neuroscientific theories but also fosters the translation of fundamental research into clinical and technological innovations, reinforcing the reciprocal interplay between brain science and artificial intelligence.

Contemporary neuroscience has progressed beyond the traditional framework of localized functional mapping, which sought to attribute specific cognitive functions to anatomically discrete brain regions. Instead, a more integrative and dynamic perspective has emerged, one that conceptualizes the brain as a complex system of distributed and interacting neural networks

(Bassett and Sporns, 2017). In this model, cognitive processes are understood not as the product of isolated regions, but as emergent properties arising from the nonlinear and temporally coordinated interactions among multiple brain systems. These interactions span various spatial and temporal scales, encompassing fast oscillatory dynamics, regional synchronization, and large-scale network connectivity that evolves over time.

This epistemological shift has been strongly propelled by the development of advanced neurotechnologies and computational tools capable of capturing and interpreting the brain's multiscale complexity. Functional neuroimaging modalities, such as functional magnetic resonance imaging and positron emission tomography, have enabled the visualization of macroscopic patterns of brain activity, while high-resolution electrophysiological techniques, including electroencephalography and magnetoencephalography, provide access to rapid temporal dynamics of neural signaling. These complementary modalities generate large, high-dimensional datasets that reflect the brain's structural and functional organization in unprecedented detail.

To effectively interpret these data, neuroscience has increasingly turned to computational models grounded in machine learning, particularly deep learning architectures. These models excel in identifying latent representations within complex signals, learning hierarchical structures, and extracting features that may be difficult to detect through conventional statistical methods. Deep neural networks, in particular, are capable of capturing both spatial and temporal dependencies in neural data, thereby offering insights into the mechanisms by which information is processed, integrated, and transmitted across brain circuits (Ju and Bassett, 2020). Moreover, their ability to generalize across data from different individuals and experimental contexts positions them as powerful tools for uncovering neurobiological principles that are robust and scalable (Mastrogiuseppe et al., 2022).

Consequently, computational intelligence has become a central component of contemporary brain science, serving not only as an analytic tool but also as a theoretical bridge between raw empirical data and the formulation of explanatory models. This convergence of neuroscience and artificial intelligence is fostering new avenues of research aimed at decoding the fundamental principles of cognition, developing predictive models of brain function and dysfunction, and ultimately transforming our understanding of the human mind through the lens of data-driven discovery.

This chapter explores three key pillars that underpin the emerging field at the intersection of neuroscience and computational intelligence: (1) the structural and functional principles of the human brain, (2) electroencephalography (EEG) as a non-invasive tool for analyzing real-time neural dynamics, and

(3) computational methods, focusing on machine learning (ML) and deep neural networks applied to brain activity modeling. The chapter adopts an integrative perspective, emphasizing how these domains interact to deepen our understanding of brain processes and enable new applications in brain science.

The chapter is structured in three parts. It begins with the neurobiological foundations of brain organization. Next, it examines EEG, including its physical and physiological principles and practical applications. Finally, it presents key concepts in computational intelligence, highlighting their use in interpreting neurophysiological data. Throughout, the interconnections among these areas are discussed as a way to construct a broader understanding of brain function.

In the face of growing theoretical complexity and technological advancement, integrating multiscale empirical data with computational models capable of pattern inference and prediction becomes essential. Such integration represents a major step toward a more interpretable, predictive, and translational neuroscience.

Our goal is to provide an up-to-date and critical overview of this consolidating field, encouraging the training of researchers who can navigate fluently between biological and computational domains. We believe that future innovations in cognitive science, personalized medicine, and neurotechnology will emerge precisely from this convergence.

2. Neuroscience Foundations Applied to ASD

Understanding the neurobiological mechanisms underlying ASD requires an integrated, multidisciplinary approach grounded in the foundations of contemporary neuroscience. ASD is characterized by a heterogeneous set of behavioral, cognitive, and sensory manifestations that ultimately reflect complex alterations in the development and functioning of the central nervous system. Within this context, the study of the neural bases of ASD involves the analysis of processes such as the functional organization of cerebral lobes, connectivity among neural networks, synaptic plasticity, and the dynamics of cortical oscillations. The application of knowledge from neuroscience, particularly through techniques such as electroencephalography, functional neuroimaging, and computational modeling, has enabled significant advances in the identification of neurophysiological biomarkers, the mapping of atypical neurodevelopmental trajectories, and the understanding of circuits that support social, communicative, and sensory-perceptual functions. This section outlines the key neuroscientific foundations that underpin the investigation and modeling of ASD, with emphasis on the integration of empirical data, neurocognitive theories, and analytical tools that contribute to a more accurate, predictive, and personalized approach to the disorder.

2.1 Neurofunctional Foundations of the Human Brain

The different regions of the human brain integrate into a highly complex and hierarchically organized architecture, in which multiple neural systems operate simultaneously and interdependently. This functional network combines local specializations with extensive interregional connections, enabling sensory, motor, affective, and cognitive processes to be carried out in a coordinated and adaptive manner. Structurally, the brain can be divided into distinct cortical and subcortical regions, each associated with specific functions, although human behavior emerges from the dynamic integration of these areas.

The frontal, parietal, temporal, and occipital lobes represent classical divisions of the cerebral cortex, used for both anatomical and functional purposes, reflecting the topographical distribution of tasks such as executive control, sensory perception, language, memory, emotions, and vision. Each of these regions contributes specialized subprocesses that, when integrated within a network, support higher cognitive abilities and the behavioral flexibility characteristic of the human species. However, understanding brain function requires more than mapping these specializations, it demands the examination of functional and structural connections that enable interregional communication, as well as an understanding of the mechanisms that regulate the temporal modulation of neural activity across different contexts.

Beyond anatomical subdivisions, the brain operates through distributed, dynamic circuits whose activity is regulated by mechanisms of synchrony, synaptic plasticity, and recurrent feedback. These circuits are responsible for coordinating perception, action, emotion, and thought, and are shaped by both genetic factors and lived experience. The emergence of complex cognitive functions such as consciousness, language, empathy, and prospective planning, therefore, depends on the continuous interaction between specialized regions and the central nervous system's capacity to adapt to new environmental demands throughout development and adulthood.

This integrative perspective, which considers both local specialization and functional interdependence among distant regions, has underpinned contemporary approaches in neuroscience, particularly those aimed at understanding neurodevelopmental disorders, where functional disorganization of these networks can compromise essential aspects of behavior and cognition.

The frontal lobe, located in the anterior portion of the brain, represents one of the most evolutionary recent and functionally complex regions of the human brain. It is often referred to as the "executive center" of cortical activity due to its central role in mediating higher-order processes that support decision-making, strategic planning, abstract reasoning, and behavioral regulation. This region houses the primary motor cortex, responsible for the execution of voluntary movements through direct activation of motor neurons, as well as premotor and supplementary motor areas involved in movement planning, coordination, and the automatization of motor sequences.

However, it is in the prefrontal cortex that the most notable functional complexity of the frontal lobe resides. Structurally, this region is subdivided into dorsolateral, ventromedial, and orbitofrontal domains, each associated with distinct neurofunctional circuits and specific domains of cognition and behavior. The dorsolateral prefrontal cortex, for instance, is closely involved in working memory, the manipulation of information in real time, and the modulation of attentional focus. The ventromedial prefrontal cortex, in turn, plays a key role in affective processing and the integration of emotion with cognition, influencing social and moral decision-making. Meanwhile, the orbitofrontal cortex critically contributes to the evaluation of rewards and punishments, adaptive behavior, and the inhibition of impulsive responses in social contexts.

These prefrontal systems do not operate in isolation but are functionally integrated with subcortical structures such as the thalamus, ventral striatum, amygdala, and hippocampus, forming cortico-subcortical circuits that regulate a wide range of functions, from motivated behavior to moral judgment and ethical decision-making. This functional architecture makes the frontal lobe an essential component of behavioral adaptation, emotional regulation, and the mediation of complex social interactions.

Damage to this region can result in severe neuropsychological syndromes, such as dysexecutive syndrome, characterized by difficulties in initiating and maintaining goals, perseverative behaviors, impulsiveness, and impaired social judgment. As noted by Stuss (2011), these changes compromise not only cognitive performance on laboratory tasks but also functional competence in real-world contexts, including interpersonal relationships and the workplace. Moreover, prefrontal dysfunction has been implicated in the pathophysiology of several neuropsychiatric disorders, such as attention-deficit/hyperactivity disorder (ADHD), personality disorders, schizophrenia, affective disorders, and ASD, highlighting the clinical relevance of this region to mental health.

Finally, the development of the frontal lobe occurs over an extended period throughout the lifespan, continuing into the third decade of life, with gradual synaptic maturation and myelination. This characteristic confers high plasticity but also increased vulnerability to environmental influences during neurodevelopment, making this region particularly sensitive to early adverse or enriching experiences. Thus, the study of the frontal lobe is essential for understanding the neural foundations of human cognition, social behavior, and mental health.

Frontal lobe development is relatively delayed compared to other cortical regions, achieving structural maturity only around the third decade of life. This protracted maturation has direct implications for neurodevelopment and decision-making processes during adolescence. From an electrophysiological perspective, this region exhibits theta and gamma activity particularly associated with cognitive control tasks, and its dysfunction is implicated in a wide range of neuropsychiatric disorders, including ADHD, schizophrenia, mood disorders, and autism.

The parietal lobe, located in the upper portion of the brain between the frontal and occipital lobes, plays a central role in mediating conscious sensory perception, constructing spatial cognition, and integrating multimodal sensory information. This cortical region is functionally segmented into primary and associative areas, reflecting the hierarchy of sensory processing, from elementary encoding to the formation of abstract representations of the body and space. The postcentral gyrus, corresponding to Brodmann areas 3, 1, and 2, constitutes the primary somatosensory cortex and serves as the first cortical destination for tactile afferents arriving at the brain from thalamic nuclei. Within this region, a topographic map of bodily sensations is established, enabling precise coding of the location, intensity, texture, and quality of tactile stimuli (Gottlieb and Snyder, 2010).

In addition to its primary sensory function, the parietal lobe contains posterior regions such as the superior and inferior parietal cortex, which play crucial roles in visuospatial orientation, selective attention, and sensorimotor integration. These regions are involved in constructing cognitive maps of extra personal space, which are essential for navigation, goal-directed motor coordination, and object manipulation. In particular, the superior parietal cortex contributes to the generation of motor commands mediated by spatial perception, while the inferior parietal cortex, including the supramarginal and angular gyri, is engaged in symbolic and linguistic processes such as reading, writing, mathematical calculation, and the semantic understanding of spatial and causal relationships.

From a functional perspective, the parietal lobe operates as an interface between sensory and motor systems, integrating auditory, visual, and somatosensory signals into coherent representations that guide goal-directed behavior. This intermodal integration is essential for pattern recognition in the environment and for constructing bodily awareness, mediated by circuits involving connections with the frontal lobe, basal ganglia, cerebellum, and temporal structures. Moreover, the parietal lobe supports top-down spatial attention, enabling the voluntary selection of relevant stimuli and the inhibition of distracting ones through its interaction with the dorsal attention network.

Parietal dysfunction gives rise to a range of varied and highly specific clinical syndromes that illustrate the region's functional sophistication. Lesions in the dominant hemisphere can result in Gerstmann syndrome, characterized by acalculia, agraphia, left–right disorientation, and finger agnosia, while lesions in the non-dominant hemisphere are associated with hemi spatial neglect, constructive apraxia, and disturbances in body perception (somatognosia). Additionally, conditions such as spatial agnosia and cortical ballism highlight the importance of the parietal lobe in motor orientation and three-dimensional perception.

From a developmental perspective, the parietal lobe exhibits remarkable plasticity throughout childhood and adolescence, a period during which visuospatial and mathematical skills are acquired and refined. The functional maturation of these regions is directly linked to academic performance and the development of symbolic abilities, and is influenced by genetic, environmental, and educational factors.

Thus, the parietal lobe is considered a key structure in sensory integration, motor planning, attentional orientation, and the construction of abstract representations, positioning itself as an essential functional hub for adaptive human behavior. A deeper understanding of its functions and associated circuits has significant implications for both clinical neuropsychology and neuroscience applications in education and rehabilitation.

The temporal lobe, located in the lateral portions of the brain beneath the Sylvian fissure, constitutes one of the most multifunctional and highly interconnected cortical regions of the brain, playing key roles in multiple domains of human cognition. This lobe contains both cortical and subcortical structures actively involved in auditory processing, language decoding, episodic memory, emotional regulation, and the recognition of complex patterns such as faces and objects. Functional segmentation of the temporal lobe includes the superior, middle, and inferior temporal gyri, as well as highly specialized medial structures, including the hippocampus, parahippocampal gyrus, and amygdala, all of which are fundamental components of the limbic system. The superior temporal gyrus, particularly its posterior portion in the dominant hemisphere, houses Wernicke's area, classically associated with the comprehension of spoken and written language (Wani, 2024). This region plays a crucial role in the semantic and syntactic analysis of language and is highly connected to other language areas, such as the inferior frontal gyrus (Broca's area), via the arcuate fasciculus. Lesions in this area can result in Wernicke's aphasia, characterized by fluent but meaningless speech production and severe difficulty in verbal comprehension, illustrating the functional specificity of this temporal region.

The middle temporal gyrus participates in broader semantic functions and integrates auditory information with visual and mnemonic content, playing an important role in understanding the meaning of words, objects, and social contexts. The inferior temporal gyrus, involved in visual recognition and categorization of complex stimuli, interacts with the occipitotemporal cortex (including the fusiform gyrus), contributing to face recognition, a fundamental process for social and affective cognition (Jefferies et al., 2016; Panikratova et al., 2025).

On the medial surface of the temporal lobe lies the limbic system, whose primary mnemonic structure, the hippocampus, is directly involved in the consolidation of long-term declarative memory, spatial navigation, and relational learning. The hippocampus functions as an integrative hub between cortical inputs and subcortical structures, modulating the transfer of information from the entorhinal cortex to broader neocortical regions.

In turn, the amygdala, which is closely connected to the hippocampus and hypothalamus, plays a key role in the emotional encoding of memory, affective evaluation of stimuli, and the mediation of autonomic responses to stress. Both structures are crucial for the formation of meaningful memories and are modulated by neurotransmitters such as glutamate, dopamine, and norepinephrine.

The vulnerability of the temporal lobe to various neurological conditions is well documented. Temporal lobe epilepsy is one of the most common and refractory forms of focal epilepsy, often associated with hippocampal sclerosis, emotional disturbances, and memory deficits. Alzheimer's disease typically begins with early synaptic degeneration and beta-amyloid accumulation in the entorhinal and hippocampal regions, leading to disruption of episodic memory and spatial disorientation. Traumatic brain injuries, particularly those involving rotational movements or impact at the base of the skull, also affect these vulnerable structures, resulting in mnemonic impairments and behavioral changes (Dharshini et al., 2019).

Functional and structural neuroimaging has confirmed the centrality of the temporal lobe within high-level brain networks, such as the default mode network, which is associated with introspective processes, and the limbic-cortical network, which modulates emotional responses. Alterations in the activation and connectivity of these regions have been observed in various neuropsychiatric disorders, including autism, schizophrenia, major depression, and anxiety disorders, highlighting the integrative and modulatory role of the temporal lobe in cerebral neurodynamic.

Thus, the temporal lobe emerges as a neurofunctionally dense and multifaceted region, whose integrity is essential for maintaining the communicative, affective, and mnemonic functions that underpin the human experience. Its detailed study provides valuable insights into the neural mechanisms involved in language, memory, and social cognition, while offering critical foundations for the development of therapeutic approaches in complex neurological and psychiatric conditions.

The occipital lobe, located in the most posterior portion of the brain, although smaller in anatomical extent compared to other cortical lobes, constitutes a region of extremely high functional specialization, playing a fundamental role in visual information processing. Its primary visual cortex, known as V1 or Brodmann area 17, receives direct projections from the lateral geniculate nucleus of the thalamus, which in turn relays signals originating from the retina. This area performs the initial processing of basic visual stimulus attributes, such as orientation, contrast, spatial location, and spatial frequency. From V1, the information is transmitted to secondary and tertiary visual areas (such as V2, V3, V4, and V5/MT), located mainly within the occipital lobe and partially extending into the parietal and temporal lobes, forming a functional hierarchy that underpins the complexity of human visual perception (Palejwala et al., 2021).

From a functional perspective, two major cortical pathways are responsible for processing visual information: the dorsal stream, which projects to the posterior parietal lobe and is involved in analyzing the spatial location, motion, and orientation of objects in the environment; and the ventral stream, which extends toward the inferior temporal lobe and is responsible for object, face, and complex visual pattern recognition. This functional duality, widely known as the "two-stream model", constitutes one of the foundational frameworks of contemporary visual neuroscience, supported by extensive neuroanatomical literature as well as studies using functional neuroimaging and brain lesion analyses (Vaziri-Pashkam and Xu, 2017).

The proper functioning of the occipital lobe is essential for constructing a coherent visual experience, as alterations at any level of this system can severely compromise perception. Bilateral lesions in V1, for example, result in cortical blindness, a condition in which the patient is unable to consciously perceive visual stimuli, although subcortical structures such as the superior colliculus may still mediate reflexive responses to light, a phenomenon known as 'blindsight'. Lesions in the ventral stream can lead to prosopagnosia, a specific deficit in face recognition despite otherwise preserved visual function. In contrast, lesions affecting the dorsal stream are associated with syndromes such as Balint's syndrome, characterized by optic ataxia, ocular apraxia, and simultanagnosia (Azzopardi and Cowey, 1997; Bittar et al., 1999).

In addition to acquired lesions, neurodevelopmental disorders can also affect occipital functions. Evidence suggests that alterations in occipital networks are associated with ASD, visual dyslexia, and certain types of developmental agnosia. Structural and functional neuroimaging studies show that individuals with these conditions exhibit atypical patterns of connectivity and activation in the visual cortex, indicating that the anatomical and functional integrity of the occipital lobe is essential not only for sensory perception but also for higher cognitive processes such as language, memory, and social cognition.

From this perspective, a detailed understanding of the anatomical and functional organization of the occipital lobe, as well as its connections with other cortical and subcortical regions, is essential for advancing neuroscience knowledge regarding visual perception and its clinical implications. This integrative approach has enabled the development of more effective therapeutic and rehabilitative interventions grounded in precise neurofunctional evidence.

Understanding the neurofunctional foundations of the human brain is indispensable for advancing the sciences of behavior, cognition, and emotion. The integrated analysis of cerebral lobes and their respective functional networks provides theoretical and empirical support to elucidate the mechanisms by which the central nervous system regulates environmental interaction, the construction of subjectivity, and behavioral adaptation. Investigating the dynamics of connectivity between cortical and subcortical regions, mediated by oscillatory patterns and synaptic plasticity mechanisms, reveals the complexity and sophistication of the brain as an adaptive system highly sensitive to genetic, epigenetic, and environmental influences.

This perspective, which integrates regional specialization with network-level connectivity, has direct implications for understanding atypical brain function profiles observed in various clinical contexts. Building on these foundations, it becomes possible to investigate how alterations in specific neural circuits may impact the development of cognitive and socioemotional skills, a topic that will be explored in greater depth in the following section.

2.2 *Typical Brain Development vs. ASD Neurodevelopment*

Human neurodevelopment is a multifaceted, progressive process that critically depends on dynamic interactions among genetic, epigenetic, and environmental factors, which shape the structure and functionality of the central nervous system over time. From early embryonic stages, the brain undergoes critical events such as neural proliferation, cell migration, neuronal differentiation, synaptogenesis, myelination, and synaptic pruning, all of which occur according to a precise and coordinated chronology (Hadders-Algra, 2018). This sequential progression enables the gradual emergence of integrated neural networks capable of supporting the complex cognitive, emotional, sensorimotor, and social functions that characterize the human species.

In typical development, the refinement of these networks follows consistent ontogenetic patterns. During childhood and adolescence, progressive functional specialization occurs, mediated by a balance between local and global connectivity, which facilitates the strengthening of long-range circuits responsible for higher-order cognition, such as self-regulation, language, empathy, and planning (Niu et al., 2018). The efficiency of these networks is largely attributable to the maturation of white matter and the reorganization of cerebral electrical activity, marked by increased oscillatory synchrony among distributed regions (Park et al., 2020). Neural oscillation patterns, particularly in the theta, alpha, and gamma frequency bands, become increasingly stable and functionally modulated, endowing the brain with an adaptive network architecture capable of flexibly responding to environmental demands.

In contrast, ASD is characterized by marked and early deviations from this neurodevelopmental trajectory, which are not limited to quantitative delays but involve qualitative alterations in mechanisms of brain connectivity and integration (Mohammad-Rezazadeh et al., 2016). Numerous studies have identified an atypical pattern of brain growth during the first years of life in individuals with ASD, featuring early volumetric enlargement, particularly in the frontal and temporal cortex, followed by a plateau or reduction in brain volume during late childhood. This anomalous growth is frequently associated with excessive synaptic proliferation that is not accompanied by effective synaptic pruning, compromising neural network efficiency and contributing to the local hyperconnectivity observed in various neuroimaging findings (Nordahl et al., 2020; Ruan et al., 2024).

These anatomical alterations coexist with equally atypical functional patterns. Contemporary neuroscience literature highlights reduced functional connectivity among long-range networks, such as the default mode network, the salience network, and the frontoparietal network, while hyperconnectivity is observed in local circuits, particularly in primary sensory and associative regions (Jahedi et al., 2016; Shao et al., 2024). This pattern suggests a fragmented and less integrative neural organization, which may explain both behavioral rigidity and difficulties in information generalization frequently observed in ASD. Furthermore, abnormalities in the functioning of neurotransmitter systems, including GABAergic, glutamatergic, and serotonergic systems, lead to an imbalance in cortical excitability and synaptic plasticity, affecting the autistic brain's ability to modulate responses to social and sensory stimuli.

In the domain of neural oscillations, individuals with ASD exhibit distinctive electrophysiological signatures, such as reduced power and coherence of alpha rhythms during resting states, altered theta desynchronization patterns during memory tasks, and inconsistencies in gamma-band modulation during sensory and social processing (Roberts et al., 2012). These oscillations are essential for establishing communication between distant neuronal populations through a mechanism known as phase coupling. Their dysfunction, therefore, compromises the interregional integration necessary for the simultaneous processing of multiple sources of information, which may underlie the communication difficulties, impairments in shared attention, and deficits in social cognition that are characteristic of the autistic spectrum.

Moreover, connectomic studies and computational modeling have revealed specific patterns in the brain network topology of individuals with ASD, including reduced modularity, centrality, and global efficiency (Freitag et al., 2021; Liu et al., 2021). This suggests a diminished capacity for functional adaptation during complex tasks and transitions between cognitive states, directly impacting behavioral flexibility. These findings support the hypothesis that ASD does not represent a focal lesion or a unitary syndrome, but rather a condition of global brain dysrhythmia in development, characterized by failures in mechanisms of information integration and coordination across distributed networks.

From a neuropsychological development perspective, this atypical brain organization manifests early through detectable behavioral patterns within the first year of life, such as lack of communication, difficulties in maintaining eye contact, exaggerated or absent responses to sensory stimuli, and stereotyped motor patterns. Throughout development, these signs consolidate into persistent deficits in areas of reciprocal social communication, theory of mind, empathy, and cognitive flexibility, all functions supported by frontotemporal networks that exhibit atypical connectivity and activation in ASD.

Therefore, the comparison between typical brain development and the patterns observed in ASD reveals profound discrepancies in how the brain organizes its functional networks over time. Understanding these deviations, in their origin, manifestation, and trajectory, is essential for advancing early diagnostic strategies, neuroplasticity-based interventions, and theoretical frameworks that acknowledge the complexity and heterogeneity of the autistic spectrum. From this perspective, the autistic brain should not be viewed as a less functional brain, but rather as a system that organizes itself according to its own principles, requiring scientific and clinical approaches that are equally specific and tailored.

3. Basic Concepts of Electroencephalography (EEG)

EEG is a widely used non-invasive technique for recording the brain's electrical activity through electrodes placed on the scalp. These electrodes detect electrical potential generated by cortical neuronal activity, allowing real-time acquisition of brain oscillations associated with various cognitive, sensory, and motor states (Paszkiel, 2019). The electrical signals recorded by EEG are primarily produced by the synchronized activity of large populations of neurons, particularly pyramidal neurons located in the cerebral cortex. The activation of these neurons generates electrical currents resulting from the flow of ions such as sodium ($Na+$), potassium ($K+$), calcium ($Ca2+$), and chloride (Cl^-) across cell membranes (Teplan et al., 2002). These currents produce extracellular potentials that can be detected by electrodes placed on the surface of the scalp.

After acquisition, the signals are amplified and displayed as graphical tracings, known as electroencephalograms, which represent the oscillatory patterns of the brain's bioelectrical activity. This approach provides detailed insights into brain function and is particularly useful for identifying neurological abnormalities.

The technique enables precise analysis of brain activity patterns in different physiological and cognitive states, such as wakefulness, sleep, attention, and stimulus reactivity (Vecchio et al., 2014). In addition to its high temporal resolution, EEG offers the advantages of being safe, portable, and well tolerated by patients, making it an essential tool for clinical applications and neuroscience research. Its use is essential for exploring and understanding neurological and psychiatric disorders, including epilepsy, sleep disorders, and neurodevelopmental conditions such as ASD.

To ensure standardization and reproducibility in electroencephalographic measurements, electrodes are typically positioned according to the international 10–20 system. This system arranges 21 electrodes based on proportional percentages of the distance between four anatomical reference points on the skull: the nasion, inion, and left and right pre-auricular points. The letters assigned to the electrodes indicate the underlying brain regions: F (frontal), T (temporal), C (central), P (parietal), and O (occipital). Odd numbers correspond to the left hemisphere, while even numbers denote the right hemisphere. Electrodes positioned along the midline are labeled with the designation 'z' (for 'zero'), such as Fz, Cz, or Pz (Gomes et al., 2023; Homan et al., 1987).

This standardization ensures adequate topographic coverage of key cortical regions, enabling reliable comparisons between individuals and recordings, while facilitating the application of quantitative methods and brain mapping techniques.

Two fundamental parameters for interpreting electroencephalograms are the frequency and amplitude of the recorded signals. Under normal physiological conditions, the amplitude of EEG signals typically ranges between 15–150 μV, with average values between 30–80 μV. These amplitudes reflect the characteristic bioelectric activity of the brain and can vary significantly depending on the individual's mental and physiological state, such as during relaxation, concentration or sleep (Naydenov et al., 2022). Frequency represents the rhythm of brain activity and is associated with different mental and behavioral states. Traditionally, these frequencies are grouped into distinct bands: delta (0.5–4 Hz), theta (4–7 Hz), alpha (8–12 Hz), beta (13–31 Hz), and gamma (32–90 Hz), each linked to specific neurophysiological functions (Attar, 2022).

However, due to the low amplitude of signals generated by brain electrical activity, direct and accurate recording is only possible with appropriate technical resources. In this context, amplifiers play a crucial role in enhancing captured signals, ensuring recording precision and enabling more detailed and reliable analyzes (Zarifi et al., 2011).

One of the main advantages of electroencephalography is its exceptional temporal resolution, allowing the detection of brain activity fluctuations at the millisecond scale. This characteristic makes EEG particularly effective for investigating dynamic and short-lived neural processes, distinguishing it from other neuroimaging modalities such as functional magnetic resonance imaging (fMRI) and positron emission tomography (PET), which offer high spatial resolution but comparatively lower temporal precision.

In addition to its temporal resolution, EEG offers several other advantages, including equipment portability, low operational costs, ease of administration, and absence of side effects. These attributes make EEG a viable and scalable option for use in hospitals, outpatient clinics and large-scale screening programs. Recent studies highlight EEG not only as an effective diagnostic tool but also as an economically accessible, with demonstrated utility in detecting neurologically subtle abnormalities that are clinically difficult to identify, such as non-convulsive seizures and subtle brain dysfunctions (Alvi et al., 2022).

Another key consideration is EEG's cost-effectiveness, particularly in public health contexts and resource-limited settings. According to (McLane et al., 2015), the availability of diagnostic tests such as EEG is directly correlated with national income levels and healthcare infrastructure. In lower-income regions, access to advanced neuroimaging techniques such as fMRI and PET is often limited, underscoring the strategic importance of EEG in these settings.

The relatively accessible nature of electroencephalography helps expand access to high-quality neurophysiological tests, enabling earlier and more accurate diagnoses, particularly in vulnerable populations. This underscores the value of EEG in diverse settings, including remote regions, underserved urban areas, and public health initiatives in developing countries.

Despite its numerous advantages, the technique has significant limitations. The propagation of electrical signals to external electrodes requires passage through multiple biological layers, including brain tissue, cerebrospinal fluid, skull bone, and scalp, which can attenuate and distort signals. This compromises spatial resolution and makes the precise localization of electrical activity sources challenging.

EEG is highly susceptible to artifacts, including those generated by muscle movements, eye blinks, and environmental interference. Consequently, signal processing requires sophisticated preprocessing and analysis methods, and results may be affected by inter-individual variability and methodological biases, necessitating careful interpretation of findings.

Nevertheless, electroencephalography remains a vital and widely used tool, particularly in contexts where portability, low cost, safety, and high temporal resolution are critical factors, such as in neurodevelopmental studies and clinical screenings for children with suspected ASD.

In summary, electroencephalography stands as an indispensable tool for investigating brain electrical activity, providing valuable insights into a wide spectrum of mental states and neurophysiological processes. While challenges remain regarding accessibility and technical limitations, its effectiveness in detecting neurological abnormalities and assessing brain function continues to be widely recognized, solidifying its strategic role in both clinical practice and neuroscience research.

4. Fundamentals of Computational Intelligence

In this section, we present the theoretical and conceptual foundations that structure the field of Computational Intelligence (CI), understood as an interdisciplinary domain that integrates contributions from computer science, applied mathematics, computational neuroscience, statistics, and complex dynamical systems theory. CI constitutes a computational paradigm focused on building artificial systems capable of handling uncertainties, learning from data, adapting to environmental changes, and generalizing from prior experiences.

Throughout this section, we will discuss the main pillars that support this field, with emphasis on the concepts of CI, on ML techniques, and on the architectures of Artificial Neural Networks (ANNs) and Deep Neural

Networks, which represent a significant evolution in pattern processing and recognition in large volumes of data.

4.1 Concepts of Computational Intelligence

CI establishes itself as a dynamic and interdisciplinary subfield within Artificial Intelligence, focused on the design and development of sophisticated computational systems and algorithms capable of simulating fundamental aspects of human reasoning (Ojanguren, 2018). This simulation proves particularly relevant in contexts characterized by high uncertainty, imprecision, conceptual ambiguity, or complexity inherent to traditional mathematical modeling. Such conditions are common in real-world environments, where data may be incomplete, noisy, heterogeneous, or even partially contradictory, hindering the application of deterministic models based on fixed rules or rigid formal logic. In this scenario, CI proposes an alternative approach, favoring adaptive and heuristic methods that, through learning from experience, can dynamically adjust to varied and not previously defined patterns. This methodological flexibility, which enables the efficient handling of imperfect and unstructured information, has been fundamental to the advancement of CI, making it a promising tool in domains where the rigidity of conventional models proves insufficient or inadequate.

Within this broad spectrum, the main techniques of CI stand out as artificial neural networks, evolutionary algorithms, fuzzy systems, and more recently, hybrid methods that integrate and combine multiple strategies to optimize performance and robustness. ANNs inspired by the structure and functioning of the human brain, perform parallel and distributed processing, enabling the recognition and classification of complex patterns (Eberhart, 2007). These models are particularly effective in the automatic extraction of features from raw data, a property that becomes especially relevant in the processing of biomedical signals, where feature engineering is a critical and challenging step. Evolutionary algorithms are based on the principles of natural selection and biological adaptation, applying mechanisms of mutation, recombination, and selection to solve optimization problems (Deb, 2001). These algorithms offer robust search strategies in multidimensional and multimodal spaces, proving to be efficient in situations where the objective functions are discontinuous, non-differentiable, or not explicitly known. Fuzzy systems, in turn, incorporate approximate logic capable of handling the ambiguity and imprecision typical of human reasoning, bringing decision-making closer to the natural behavior of human experts (Gottwald, 2005). These systems allow for more intuitive modeling of processes where clear thresholds and binary classifications are insufficient to capture the complexity of human perceptions or physiological signals. Hybrid methods represent a recent evolution in which different CI paradigms are synergistically combined to overcome individual limitations and expand the scope of applications (Arun et al., 2024). These integrated approaches seek to combine the learning capacity of neural networks, the search efficiency of evolutionary algorithms, and the interpretability of fuzzy systems, enhancing both performance and explainability in real-world applications.

This bioinspired foundation gives CI techniques a high degree of robustness, adaptability, and generalization capacity, attributes that are indispensable in scenarios where biological variability, data ambiguity, and the absence of explicit mathematical models pose substantial challenges to computational modeling and analysis. Moreover, the intrinsic capability of CI systems to learn from examples and generalize to new situations aligns with the nature of biomedical and clinical data, which are often characterized by high inter-individual variability, evolving patterns over time, and a significant presence of noise and artifacts.

The effectiveness of CI applications has been widely demonstrated across various complex problems where traditional approaches fail or show significant limitations. Particularly in Biomedical Engineering, numerous studies have explored CI techniques for analyzing electrophysiological signals to diagnose neurological disorders. For instance, recent research investigates advanced EEG signal analysis methods for early diagnosis of ASD, demonstrating the capability of these approaches to address practical challenges – such as missing signals in some patients – without compromising the identification of neural patterns associated with the disorder (Silva, 2024). These approaches not only enable the classification of individuals based on neural activity but also contribute to the understanding of atypical brain connectivity and signal complexity patterns that may underlie the disorder. Similarly, other studies propose representing EEG signals as images for Alzheimer's diagnosis, employing Deep Learning techniques combined with interpretability methods to ensure model explainability and enhance clinical confidence in automated decisions (Souza, 2025). The use of image-based representations, such as time-frequency maps or recurrence plots, allows convolutional neural networks to explore spatial features from temporal data, enhancing diagnostic accuracy in neurodegenerative diseases.

These initiatives illustrate CI's versatility and impact in extracting clinically relevant information from complex biomedical data, contributing to significant advances in more precise and personalized diagnostics. By enabling the identification of latent structures, nonlinear relationships, and subtle patterns often imperceptible to human observers or traditional analytical methods, CI becomes an indispensable ally in precision medicine and digital health initiatives. Moreover, the capacity to integrate multimodal data, combining signals, images, clinical annotations, and demographic variables, enhances the ecological validity and translational potential of these approaches in real-world healthcare settings.

Furthermore, the application of CI has proven particularly effective in other biomedical challenges, such as automatic recognition of visual and auditory patterns, prediction of physiological time series, control of non-linear dynamic systems, and optimization of clinical processes (Sadeghi-Naini et al., 2020). In tasks such as heart rate variability analysis, seizure prediction, and motor intention decoding for brain-computer interfaces, CI methods have demonstrated superior performance in terms of sensitivity, specificity, and robustness under noisy conditions. In hospital management and logistics, evolutionary and swarm intelligence algorithms have been employed for scheduling optimization, patient flow modeling, and resource allocation, evidencing the broad applicability of CI beyond the confines of signal analysis.

Technological advances increased computational capacity, and the growing availability of large volumes of data from biomedical sensors, electronic health records, and wearable devices have driven the consolidation of CI as a central approach in strategic areas of digital health, industrial automation, financial markets, and data science. Its ability to extract latent structures and regularities from heterogeneous and noisy datasets has significantly expanded its impact on the development of innovative and cutting-edge technological solutions. In the context of healthcare, this evolution aligns with the global movement toward predictive, preventive, personalized, and participatory (P4) medicine, in which intelligent systems capable of continuous learning and adaptation play a central role. The synergistic interaction between computational models and clinical practice has the potential to transform diagnosis, monitoring, and therapeutic decision-making processes, improving not only outcomes but also the efficiency and equity of healthcare delivery systems (Zapirain et al., 2019).

4.2 Machine Learning Paradigms and Their Applications in Healthcare

The exponential advancement of information technologies and the increasing availability of large-scale data have driven the adoption of ML in the healthcare field, establishing this area as one of the most promising at the intersection of data science and biomedicine. This computational approach enables the development of algorithms capable of learning complex patterns directly from data, without the need to program explicit rules or rely on conventional statistical modeling. This feature facilitates the identification of non-trivial correlations, often imperceptible to human clinical reasoning, and leads to significant improvements in the accuracy and efficiency of diagnostic, prognostic, and therapeutic processes.

The applicability of ML in contemporary medicine ranges from the analysis of radiological images and physiological signals to the prediction of risk for multifactorial diseases, the discovery of biomarkers, and the personalization of treatments. Furthermore, ML models demonstrate generalization capability, that is, they can apply learned knowledge to new data, provided the training sample is sufficiently representative of the clinical phenomenon under study.

The main paradigms of ML include supervised learning, unsupervised learning, and reinforcement learning, each with distinct methodological characteristics and potential applications. Supervised learning is widely used in classification and regression tasks, as it involves training models using labeled examples, such as in automated diagnosis based on laboratory tests or medical imaging. Unsupervised learning, in contrast, explores unlabeled datasets to identify clusters, latent patterns, or hidden structures, making it especially valuable in exploratory studies and patient profile segmentation. Reinforcement learning is inspired by mechanisms of sequential decision-making and learning through trial and error. It has been applied in the development of autonomous agents for controlling smart medical devices, dynamic treatment management, and adaptive clinical simulations.

In this section, the conceptual foundations of each paradigm are presented, along with their epistemological implications, technical limitations, and applications within the biomedical context. Particular emphasis is placed on the use of ML in predictive, classificatory, and adaptive tasks, aligned with the demands of an increasingly data-driven, personalized, and patient-centered medicine, without overlooking ethical principles, model interpretability, and the regulatory challenges inherent to its clinical implementation.

ML, one of the foundational pillars of Artificial Intelligence, comprises a set of computational methods that enable systems to recognize complex patterns in large volumes of data, perform inferences, and improve their performance in specific tasks based on accumulated experience, without the need for explicit programming for each particular situation (El Naqa and Murphy, 2015; Hahn, 2019). This approach represents a paradigm shift in the design of computational systems, moving the focus from traditional deterministic programming toward data-driven statistical modeling. Rather than relying on pre-defined instructions provided by human experts, ML algorithms learn directly from presented examples, adjusting their internal parameters based on feedback derived from the data.

This learning process is grounded in mathematical and statistical principles, including concepts from optimization, linear algebra, information theory, and probability, which endow models with adaptive capacity, robustness, and generalization. Consequently, when exposed to new data, these systems are able to make predictions, classifications, or recommendations based on previously identified patterns, even in high-dimensional, noisy, or uncertain contexts. This capability is particularly relevant in the biomedical domain, where data are often heterogeneous, complex, and derived from multiple sources, such as medical images, electronic health records, laboratory tests, physiological sensors, and genomic data.

The integration of ML into scientific and clinical practice has driven significant advancements in personalized medicine, early disease detection, risk stratification, and the development of more effective therapeutic interventions. Furthermore, its application extends to clinical decision-support systems, assistive robotics, drug development, and continuous health monitoring, fostering a new paradigm based on the integration of medical knowledge and computational intelligence. However, the ethical, transparent, and reliable use of these systems requires rigorous attention to issues such as model interpretability, algorithmic bias, data privacy, and external validation, in order to ensure their safe and responsible implementation in sensitive environments such as healthcare.

In the biomedical domain, ML has demonstrated substantial potential by automating and optimizing clinical and diagnostic processes that have traditionally relied on specialized human evaluation. This has led to significant advancements in terms of accuracy, scalability, and operational efficiency, particularly in areas such as medical image analysis, prediction of clinical outcomes, identification of patterns in physiological signals, and clinical decision support (El Naqa and Murphy, 2015). Methodologically, ML algorithms are typically classified into three major paradigms: supervised learning, which uses labeled datasets, where inputs are associated with known outputs, to train models capable of making predictions or classifications on new, unseen data; unsupervised learning, which aims to infer latent structures and underlying patterns in unlabeled data; and reinforcement learning, in which an agent learns through interaction with an environment, adjusting its behavior based on reward or penalty signals. The choice of the most appropriate paradigm depends on the nature of the available data and the specific objectives of the task at hand.

These distinct approaches substantially enhance the capacity for analysis and interpretation of large volumes of biomedical data, enabling the development of robust predictive models and adaptive systems. Consequently,

ML emerges as a strategic tool for knowledge generation in highly complex domains, such as personalized medicine, computational neuroscience, and artificial intelligence-assisted diagnosis.

Supervised learning constitutes the most established and widely used approach in the field of artificial intelligence. According to Singh (2019), this technique relies on algorithms that learn from pre-labeled datasets, that is, datasets in which inputs are associated with known outputs, with the goal of making predictions or classifications on new instances. This characteristic makes supervised learning particularly effective for classification tasks, in which data are organized into distinct categories based on patterns extracted from existing examples.

Studies such as those by Choudhary and Gianey (2017), and Jiang, Gradus and Rosellini (2020) highlight the importance of supervised learning in complex clinical contexts, such as mental health, where model robustness and generalization capacity are key factors in ensuring the reliability of predictive systems. In these applications, the performance of supervised models depends not only on the quality and representativeness of the input data but also on the careful selection of predictor variables and the appropriate choice of algorithms, such as support vector machines, decision trees, and artificial neural networks.

A paradigmatic application of supervised learning lies in the classification of medical images for diagnostic purposes, where algorithms are trained on datasets containing images annotated by experts, enabling systems to recognize visual patterns indicative of specific pathologies (Pereira et al., 2021; Santana et al., 2022). For instance, systems trained to detect abnormalities in X-rays or MRI scans have served as clinical decision-support tools, contributing to improved diagnostic accuracy and faster result delivery. This predictive and adaptive capability is essential for the implementation of intelligent systems in clinical settings, as it allows for continuous model refinement through the progressive incorporation of new data. As highlighted by Gomes et al. (2020), supervised learning holds transformative potential in contemporary medicine by fostering the development of data-driven solutions that enhance the precision, efficiency, and personalization of clinical decision-making processes.

Another promising application of supervised learning lies at the intersection of artificial intelligence and neuroengineering, particularly in the use of electroencephalographic (EEG) signals for classifying individuals with and without ASD. In this context, supervised algorithms are trained on labeled EEG recordings obtained from both control groups and patients diagnosed with ASD, enabling the system to learn distinctive neural patterns associated with each group. As highlighted by de Oliveira Silva et al. (2024), this methodology has demonstrated high accuracy in identifying electrophysiological biomarkers linked to the autistic spectrum, emerging as a promising complement to conventional clinical approaches. In contrast, unsupervised learning, as defined by Vermeulen (2020), refers to techniques that display functions capable of describing latent structures within unlabeled datasets. Unlike the supervised paradigm, the goal is not to establish explicit relationships between input and output variables, but rather to uncover underlying patterns and natural groupings present in the data. In the healthcare context, a relevant application of unsupervised learning lies in patient segmentation based on clinical and demographic profiles. Unsupervised algorithms are employed to group patients who share similar characteristics Espinola et al. (2021a,b), facilitating the identification of subgroups that may respond homogeneously to specific treatments.

This enables the personalization of therapeutic interventions and the optimization of clinical outcomes (Singh, 2019). By uncovering latent patterns and complex structures in biomedical data, unsupervised learning provides an innovative perspective for the individualization of medicine, contributing to significant advancements in diagnostic, prognostic, and therapeutic fields.

Finally, reinforcement learning represents a unique approach within the spectrum of ML, in which computational agents develop optimal action policies in dynamic environments by responding to reward and penalty signals (Mahajan, 2014). Unlike the supervised and unsupervised paradigms, this approach is based on the agent's continuous interaction with the environment, fostering a progressive learning process grounded in trial-and-error mechanisms.

This methodology has shown promising applications in computer vision tasks, such as object detection and recognition, where decision policies are continuously refined through accumulated experience and feedback (Bernstein and Burnaev, 2018). It stands out for its intrinsic ability to adapt in real time, a feature that makes it particularly effective in domains characterized by high complexity and unpredictability (Jhaveri et al., 2022).

The dynamic adaptability and continuous self-adjustment capability position reinforcement learning as a central approach in the development of intelligent autonomous systems, particularly in fields such as cognitive robotics and personalized medicine, where the ability to learn from the environment and adjust strategies in real time is critical for optimizing clinical outcomes.

Therefore, ML represents a paradigmatic transformation in artificial intelligence, endowing computational systems with the ability to evolve autonomously and improve their performance through experience. Its distinct approaches, supervised, unsupervised, and reinforcement learning, constitute a robust methodological spectrum capable of addressing a wide range of applications, from predictive tasks to adaptive modeling of complex environments.

In the biomedical field, ML has established itself as a strategic technology, enabling the automation of sophisticated clinical processes and driving significant advancements in diagnostic efficiency and therapeutic precision. By facilitating the analysis and interpretation of large biomedical datasets, this technology is steering medicine toward an increasingly personalized, predictive, and evidence-based model. Therefore, within a dynamic and continuously evolving scientific and technological landscape, ML emerges as one of the central pillars of innovation, fostering meaningful discoveries and redefining the paradigms of clinical practice and translational health research. The increasing adoption of ML-based methodologies in the healthcare field represents a decisive step toward precision medicine, enabling faster diagnostics, personalized treatments, and optimized use of clinical resources. As access to biomedical data expands and algorithms continue to improve, ML is expected to play an increasingly strategic role in developing intelligent solutions to contemporary medical challenges.

4.3 Artificial Neural Networks

The human brain possesses remarkable abilities developed over millions of years of evolution. We can, in fractions of a second, recognize familiar faces in a crowd, identify subtle emotional expressions, anticipate movements or the consequences of actions, and understand linguistic nuances even in noisy environments or when the speaker is not visible. These capabilities involve massive parallel processing, multimodal integration of sensory information, and a generalization ability that continues to challenge conventional computational systems.

Although these processes may seem trivial in everyday experience, they still represent a major challenge for modern computers and algorithms. Despite their advancements, such systems require large volumes of data, intensive training, and either sequential or distributed processing to achieve comparable performance on specific tasks. Even then, they often struggle to transfer learned knowledge from one context to another with the same flexibility demonstrated by the human brain.

Moreover, a remarkable feature of the brain is its neuroplasticity, that is, the ability to modify synaptic connections and reorganize neural networks in response to external stimuli, experiences, or injuries. Thanks to this plasticity, the central nervous system can acquire new skills, adapt to environmental changes, and even compensate for the loss of certain functions following structural damage, as seen in neurological rehabilitation processes after strokes or traumatic brain injuries. In contrast, computers and artificial systems rely on periodic maintenance, hardware and software updates, and component replacement when physical failures occur. A single defective component can compromise the entire operation of an electronic device, completely interrupting information processing. In the human brain, however, redundancy of circuits and reorganization capacity enable a level of resilience that remains difficult to replicate in artificial systems (Krogh, 2008).

These fundamental differences motivate interdisciplinary research in fields such as computational neuroscience, artificial intelligence, and biomedical engineering, aiming to understand how biological principles can inspire the creation of more robust, adaptive, and fault-tolerant algorithms. Thus, exploring the uniqueness of the human brain not only expands our knowledge of the mind but also drives the development of technologies that are still modest but seek to emulate its most sophisticated functions. Brain operations occur through an intricate network of billions of neurons, interconnected in a highly efficient manner, communicating via electrical impulses and chemical signals. The neuron, the basic structural and functional unit of the nervous system, consists of three main parts: the cell body (or soma), dendrites, and axon.

The dendrites are branched extensions that serve as receivers of stimuli from the environment or from other neurons. They function as biological antennas, capable of capturing and integrating thousands of signals simultaneously, contributing to the complexity and plasticity of neural networks. After reception, these signals converge toward the cell body, which houses the nucleus containing chromosomes and other essential organelles responsible for maintaining the cell's metabolic activity. The cell body performs the initial processing of the received signals, determining whether the stimulus will be transmitted further along the neuron.

The axon, in turn, is an elongated extension that transmits the nerve impulse from the cell body to other cells, whether neurons, muscle cells, or glands. Each neuron has a single axon, which can branch extensively along its path, forming terminal arborizations capable of establishing synapses with multiple target cells. This branched architecture significantly enhances the reach and efficiency of neuronal communication, allowing a single neuron to influence multiple regions of the nervous system in a coordinated and synchronized manner (Favoretto et al. 2016; Haykin, 2001).

The complexity and organization of this biological network serve as inspiration for the development of computational models in artificial intelligence, particularly artificial neural networks, which aim to emulate, albeit in a simplified manner, the cooperative functioning of biological neurons. These points of contact between neurons are called synapses, specialized structures that enable intercellular communication and play a central role in the processes of information encoding, storage, and retrieval. Thus, synapses are considered the fundamental units of neuronal interactions and are closely associated with learning capacity and memory formation.

In the adult brain, the ability to create, modify, and eliminate synapses endows the nervous system with a remarkable property known as synaptic plasticity, which serves as the neurobiological basis for behavioral and cognitive adaptation. This plasticity allows the brain to continuously reorganize itself in response to environmental stimuli, lived experiences, or structural damage, as seen in cases of trauma, injury, or neurodegenerative diseases.

Synaptic changes can manifest in various ways, including the strengthening or weakening of existing connections, the formation of new links between neurons, and, in some cases, the generation of new neurons, a phenomenon known as neurogenesis. In addition to structural modifications, the brain is capable of functionally reorganizing its neural networks, redirecting lost functions to non-lesioned areas, thereby ensuring the preservation, albeit partial, of cognitive and motor abilities.

This synaptic and functional plasticity is one of the most fascinating aspects of the human nervous system, as it ensures not only lifelong learning but also adaptive recovery in the face of clinical challenges, making the brain a uniquely resilient and versatile structure.

Building upon the functional principles of the biological neuron, McCulloch and Pitts introduced a mathematical model in 1943 that laid the foundation for the concept of the artificial neuron as the elementary unit of information processing. The artificial neuron can be described by a set of inputs $x_1, x_2, \ldots, x_n$, which simulate the electrical impulses received by the dendrites. Each input is associated with a corresponding synaptic weight $w_1, w_2, \ldots, w_n$, representing the strength of the synaptic connections in a biological neuron. These weights can take on positive values, simulating excitatory synapses, or negative values, corresponding to inhibitory synapses.

The weighted signals are then summed by an adder unit, resulting in an activation potential u. Subsequently, an activation function $g(u)$ is applied to limit the amplitude of the output signal y, which represents the response transmitted by the axon. In the biological analog, the summation unit and activation function correspond to the cell body, where processing and the generation of the action potential take place.

The original model proposed by McCulloch and Pitts has a binary nature, such that both the inputs and the output take on discrete values (typically 0 or 1), simulating in a simplified manner the firing behavior of a real neuron (Grossi and Buscema 2007; Krogh, 2008). Illustratively, the artificial neuron can be understood as a mechanism for making binary decisions (0 or 1), based on a weighted combination of evidence. Imagine, for example, a common situation in which a person must decide whether to spend the weekend at the beach. In making this decision, several factors are considered, such as weather forecast, availability of transportation, and the presence of friends for company. Each of these factors can be represented as a binary input variable in the model, simplifying how the human brain makes judgments based on multiple pieces of information.

For instance, the weather forecast can be encoded as input x_1: $x_1 = 0$ indicates rainy weather, while $x_1 = 1$ corresponds to a sunny forecast. Similarly, the availability of a car for the trip can be represented by x_2, and the presence of friends by x_3. However, each of these factors contributes differently to the final decision, reflecting the subjective weight the person assigns to each aspect. In this hypothetical scenario, the weather is of primary importance, while transportation and company are relevant but carry less weight. Therefore, weights of 7 can be assigned to the weather factor, 4 to transportation, and 2 to the presence of friends.

Next, a threshold or decision boundary is established, which determines when the outcome will favor going to the beach. Assuming this threshold is set at 5, the weighted sum of the inputs, that is, the combination of all factors, each multiplied by its respective weight, must exceed this value for the final result to be $y = 1$ (deciding to go to the beach). Otherwise, the output will be $y = 0$ (choosing to stay home). Thus, in this example, the artificial neuron operates as a linear classifier, categorizing the situation into one of two possible decisions based on objective criteria and subjective weightings. This example, although simplified, serves as an illustrative introduction to how the artificial neuron model replicates, in a basic way, the decision-making processes of biological systems. While in the human brain this integration of information occurs in parallel, massively distributed, and subject to neuromodulatory influences, in the artificial neuron it is translated into straightforward mathematical operations. This allows computational systems to learn how to classify information and make decisions when exposed to different input combinations. This principle forms the foundation of more complex models, such as artificial neural networks, which expand upon this basic structure to address problems of high complexity and large data volumes.

This artificial neuron model, also known as the Perceptron, constitutes the fundamental unit of ANNs. The Perceptron was introduced by Rosenblatt in the 1950s, building upon the earlier concepts proposed by McCulloch and

Pitts, and became a landmark in the development of more complex neural network architectures used today.

In the simplest arrangement of an ANN, known as a single-layer network, artificial neurons receive input signals directly and generate outputs without the presence of intermediate processing layers. In this type of architecture, the input layer merely acts as a distribution medium for the signals to the output layer, performing no internal processing operations.

Single-layer networks have limited representational capacity and are only capable of solving classification problems in which the classes can be separated by a linear boundary in the feature space. This limitation became evident through the contributions of Minsky and Papert in the 1960s, when they demonstrated that single-layer Perceptrons are unable to solve problems such as the XOR logical function, which cannot be linearly separated.

Despite this limitation, the Perceptron held significant historical importance as it laid the foundation for the development of more sophisticated models, such as multilayer networks. In these advanced models, the introduction of hidden layers and nonlinear activation functions enabled the overcoming of initial limitations, making it possible to solve complex problems in classification, regression, and pattern recognition.

Therefore, the study of the Perceptron and single-layer networks remains essential for understanding the foundational principles underlying modern neural architectures and for critically analyzing the training techniques that enabled major advancements in contemporary artificial intelligence Haykin (2001). Another type of ANN architecture is represented by multilayer networks. In this model, the input layer neurons distribute signals to one or more intermediate layers, also known as hidden layers. Each hidden layer consists of processing units that perform nonlinear operations on the received signals, enabling the network to learn increasingly abstract and complex representations of the input data. Communication between layers occurs in a fully interconnected manner, meaning that each neuron in one layer is connected to every neuron in the subsequent layer. This characteristic gives these architectures the name "fully connected networks", ensuring a greater capacity to model intricate patterns in the data. After processing in the hidden layers, the signals are forwarded to the output layer, which is responsible for providing the final response of the network for a given task, such as classification, regression, or pattern detection. The use of multiple hidden layers enables these networks to solve problems that cannot be addressed by single-layer networks, such as those in which the separation between classes cannot be represented by a linear boundary.

Despite their greater computational power and flexibility in capturing nonlinear relationships in data, multilayer neural networks also present additional challenges, such as increased training time, higher computational resource requirements, and the risk of overfitting when appropriate regularization and validation techniques are not applied.

Nevertheless, the development of efficient training algorithms, such as the error backpropagation method and its variants, has made the practical use of these networks in complex applications feasible, establishing them as central components in many modern artificial intelligence solutions Haykin (2001). By varying the synaptic weights and thresholds, different decision models can be obtained. In this context, the training process of an ANN consists of recursively adjusting these weights, which can be carried out in a supervised or unsupervised manner. In the former, a set of input and output data is presented to the network for training, and the weights are adjusted until the obtained output matches the expected output. In the unsupervised learning mode, on the other hand, the expected output is not provided to the network, meaning that unlabeled data is used. In this case, the goal is for the network to identify similarities and patterns among the input data, learning to distinguish them from one another. This training phase is typically the most computationally demanding in ANNs, heavily dependent on the network's architecture.

Due to this capability, ANNs are able to learn and generalize knowledge, providing appropriate responses even for situations that were not previously encountered during the training process or by the learning algorithm. This generalization ability is essential for ANNs to operate effectively in real-world environments, where data may vary and do not always exactly match the data used during training. Thus, ANNs demonstrate significant robustness and flexibility in solving complex and dynamic problems, even when the available information is noisy or incomplete.

For this reason, neural networks have been successfully applied across various sectors of society, such as in industry Alkimani et al. (2019), where they assist in process automation and predictive maintenance; in medicine Gomes et al. (2022); Shirahige et al. (2022), contributing to diagnosis, prognosis, and personalized treatment; in security Ahmadi et al. (2020), within surveillance systems and fraud detection; in education Valko and Osadchyi (2020), through the development of adaptive learning platforms; in politics Borisyuk et al. (2005), for forecasting election outcomes; and in economics Shachmurove et al. (2002), in predictive analyses of financial markets.

4.4 Deep Neural Networks

Deep neural networks have become one of the most powerful and promising approaches in the field of ML and artificial intelligence over the past few decades. The deep architecture of these networks, characterized by a large number of hidden layers, enables the learning of hierarchical and progressively abstract data representations, where each subsequent layer captures more complex and semantic information. This layered learning hierarchy is essential for effectively modeling nonlinear and complex relationships in high-dimensional spaces, an essential feature for solving challenging tasks such as pattern recognition and classification, natural language processing, time series analysis, recommendation systems, and many other applications.

Within deep architectures, Convolutional Neural Networks (CNNs) stand out due to their specialized structure that exploits intrinsic properties of spatial and temporal data. CNNs are specifically designed to leverage locality and translational invariance features commonly found in images, biomedical signals, and time sequences. This is achieved through the application of convolutional filters, which act as automatic detectors of local patterns, extracting relevant features at different levels of granularity. The incorporation of pooling layers further supports this process by reducing data dimensionality and promoting invariance to minor distortions and shifts, resulting in robust and generalizable models. Additionally, the use of regularization techniques such as dropout and normalization methods like batch normalization has been crucial in improving training stability and preventing overfitting, contributing to the continuous advancement of CNNs across multiple domains (LeCun et al., 2015). Historically, LeNet, developed by LeCun et al. in the late 1990s, marked a turning point by demonstrating the practical feasibility of using convolutional networks for real-world handwritten character recognition tasks (LeCun et al., 1998). LeNet incorporated, within a relatively simple architecture, the fundamental operations of convolution and pooling, followed by fully connected layers, establishing a pioneering model that paved the way for deeper and more complex architectures. The simplicity and efficiency of LeNet allowed its initial application in automated bank check reading systems, exemplifying its direct impact on commercial and industrial solutions.

With increased computational capacity and the availability of large-scale datasets, deeper and more complex architectures emerged, such as VGG16. This network stands out for its uniform use of 3×3 convolutional filters, enabling the extraction of more refined and detailed features, which led to substantial improvements in performance on image classification tasks. Despite its high computational demand and large number of parameters, VGG16 became a reference standard for computer vision models and has been widely used for transfer learning across different domains (Theckedath and Sedamkar, 2020).

Aiming to optimize computational efficiency and reduce model size, SqueezeNet was proposed as a lightweight and compact alternative while maintaining competitive performance comparable to larger architectures.

The core strategy of SqueezeNet involves the use of 'fire' modules, which perform a compression (squeeze) followed by an expansion (expand) of convolutional channels. This approach significantly reduces the number of parameters without meaningful loss in accuracy. This feature makes SqueezeNet particularly suitable for applications on hardware-constrained devices, such as smartphones, drones, and embedded systems, where energy efficiency and inference speed are critical factors.

A Residual Network (ResNet) introduced another fundamental innovation in the field of deep learning by revolutionizing the training of very deep networks through the concept of residual blocks with shortcut connections (Theckedath and Sedamkar, 2020). This mechanism allows the direct flow of gradients through the network, mitigating the vanishing gradient problem that traditionally hinders learning in very deep architectures. With residual connections, ResNet enables effective training of networks with hundreds of layers, an achievement previously considered unfeasible. This capability to train extremely deep models has significantly enhanced performance on complex computer vision challenges, making ResNet a landmark in deep architecture development and a foundation for numerous subsequent studies.

However, despite the considerable advancements brought by CNNs, these architectures still face significant challenges that limit their application and further development. One major limitation is the reliance on large labeled datasets to ensure model generalization. In many fields, particularly specialized domains such as medicine, acquiring large annotated datasets is difficult, costly, and time-consuming, which can constrain the applicability of CNNs. Additionally, training deep networks demands substantial computational power, often requiring advanced GPUs (graphics processing units) and long processing times, limiting access to these resources for many research groups and organizations. Furthermore, the phenomenon of overfitting remains a persistent concern, especially in scenarios involving limited or imbalanced data. When overfitting occurs, the model learns specific details and noise from the training set, compromising its ability to generalize to new data and reducing the system's practical utility. Although regularization techniques, data augmentation, and cross-validation are commonly used to mitigate this issue, they do not completely eliminate the risk of overfitting.

Another critical challenge concerns the interpretability of models, which decreases significantly as networks become deeper and more complex. The difficulty in understanding internal processes and identifying the reasons behind detected patterns or specific decisions hinders trust and adoption of these technologies in domains that require transparency, such as healthcare, finance, and security. Recent research has focused on developing explainability methods and visualization techniques for network activations, aiming to make models more interpretable and reliable. However, there is still a long way to go to achieve fully transparent and trustworthy deep learning systems.

Finally, continuous advancements in architectures, training techniques, optimization strategies, and data collection and annotation practices have driven the evolution of CNNs and deep networks, expanding their range of applications and societal impact. The convergence of artificial intelligence, data science, and domain-specific knowledge promises to transform multiple sectors, from medical diagnostics to industrial automation and human-machine interaction, reinforcing the importance of in-depth study and innovation in this field.

5. Conclusion

The integrated study of neuroscience and CI has driven significant advances in understanding the human brain by combining theoretical and technical approaches capable of exploring everything from the most basic levels of neuronal activity to complex patterns of functional organization. This convergence of disciplines allows for a comprehensive exploration of brain function, spanning multiple spatial and temporal scales, from ion channel dynamics at the cellular level to large-scale network interactions underpinning cognition and behavior. Through this interdisciplinary lens, researchers have uncovered fundamental aspects of brain structure and function, particularly emphasizing the pivotal role of distributed neural networks that facilitate efficient communication and coordination between specialized regions involved in diverse cognitive, sensory, and motor functions. These networks are characterized by their dynamic connectivity patterns, enabling flexible information processing that adapts to varying contextual demands and supports complex behaviors such as learning, memory, attention, and decision-making. Throughout this chapter, we have examined how neurobiological principles of connectivity, synaptic modulation, and brain plasticity constitute the foundational mechanisms for information processing within the nervous system, and how these principles can be effectively translated into biologically inspired computational models designed to emulate neural computation and adaptability.

Additionally, we examined the use of electroencephalography as an indispensable technique in the investigation of brain dynamics. EEG captures electrical oscillations generated by synchronized neuronal populations with exceptional temporal resolution on the order of milliseconds, making it uniquely suited to study the fast-evolving processes of neural communication. Its non-invasive nature, portability, relative affordability, and ease of deployment have established EEG as a widely accessible tool both in clinical diagnostics and experimental neuroscience research. These attributes have enabled EEG to contribute extensively to the mapping of various mental states, the identification of biomarkers related to neurological and psychiatric conditions, and the real-time monitoring of brain activity during cognitive tasks. Moreover, EEG serves as a crucial interface in BCI technologies, facilitating direct communication pathways between the brain and external devices, which holds transformative potential for neurorehabilitation, assistive technologies, and human augmentation.

Finally, we addressed the transformative role of CI within contemporary neuroscience, particularly highlighting the advancements offered by ANNs and deep learning algorithms. These computational approaches have demonstrated remarkable efficacy in processing and interpreting the large volumes of neurophysiological data that characterize modern brain research, datasets often marked by complex structures, high dimensionality, noise, and considerable interindividual variability. By leveraging sophisticated architectures capable of modeling nonlinear relationships and extracting latent representations, these techniques facilitate a more nuanced and comprehensive analysis of brain signals. Consequently, they provide a powerful foundation for constructing predictive models that simulate various aspects of human cognitive processing and neural function. For example, deep neural networks have been effectively applied in tasks such as the detection and classification of mental states, identification of pathological patterns linked to neurological disorders, and prediction of cognitive or behavioral responses to stimuli. Such applications bring the field closer to realizing functional models of brain activity, capable of supporting diagnostics, personalized medicine, and adaptive therapeutic interventions.

Moreover, the ongoing development of adaptive and predictive computational systems inspired by the principles of neural information processing opens novel possibilities for clinical and technological applications. These include the early detection and diagnosis of neurological and psychiatric disorders, the optimization of rehabilitation protocols, and the enhancement of brain-machine interfaces that allow for more seamless and intuitive interaction between humans and machines. These advancements are not only expanding the horizons of neuroengineering but are also fostering the emergence of new paradigms in human-computer interaction, where continuous feedback and learning enable systems to adapt dynamically to user needs and states.

In this context, it becomes increasingly evident that robust collaboration among neuroscientists, engineers, computer scientists, clinicians, and ethicists is essential to consolidate and propel this rapidly expanding interdisciplinary field. The establishment of integrated platforms for multimodal data analysis, the aggregation and sharing of multicenter databases to ensure data diversity and representativeness, and the development of transparent, interpretable, and ethically responsible algorithms emerge as critical priorities. These efforts aim to bridge the gap between theoretical innovation and practical application, ensuring that technological breakthroughs translate into safe, effective, and equitable solutions for healthcare and society. Furthermore, addressing ethical considerations such as data privacy, algorithmic bias, and informed consent remains fundamental in guiding responsible research and deployment of these technologies.

Thus, computational neuroscience not only advances our understanding of the mechanisms underlying the human mind but also plays a decisive role in the advent of novel diagnostic tools, rehabilitative strategies, and human-machine interaction methodologies. This confluence signals a future in which the symbiosis between brain and machine becomes increasingly tangible, promising transformative impacts across medicine, technology, and human experience.

Acknowledgement(s)

This study was financed in part by the Coordenação de Aperfeiçoamento de Pessoal de Nível Superior–Brazil (CAPES)–Finance Code 001.

Disclosure statement

The authors have no financial or non-financial conflict interests to declare.

References

Ahmadi, R., S.A.H. Shybt, et al. (2020). Study of artificial neural networks in information security risk assessment. *Journal of Management and Accounting Studies*, *8*(2), 1–10.

Alkinani, H.H., A.T. Al-Hameedi, S. Dunn-Norman, R.E. Flori, M.T. Alsaba and Amer, A.S. (2019). Applications of artificial neural networks in the petroleum industry: A review. In: *SPE Middle East Oil and Gas Show and Conference*. OnePetro.

Amunts, K., M. Migliore, A. Destexhe, L. Bitsch, J. DeFelipe, Y.E. Ioannidis, A. Knoll, R. Goebel, S. Furber, C. Pennartz, T. Lippert, M. Sanchez-Vives, V. Jirsa, J. Bjaalie and P. Ryvlin. (2022). Linking brain structure, activity, and cognitive function through computation. *eNeuro*, *9*.

Arun, C.A., P.P. Selvam, K. Deiwakumari, S.D. Govardhan, J. Jeyasudha and R. Push Pavalli. (2024). Hybrid computational intelligence models for robust pattern recognition and data analysis. *International Journal of Computational and Experimental Science and Engineering*.

Attar, E.T. (2022). A review of mental stress and EEG band power. *International Journal of Nanotechnology and Nanomedicine*.

Azzopardi, P. and A. Cowey. (1997). Is blindsight like normal, near-threshold vision? *Proceedings of the National Academy of Sciences of the United States of America*, *94* (25), 14190–14194.

Bassett, D. and O. Sporns. (2017). Network neuroscience. *Nature Neuroscience*, *20*, 353–364.

Bernstein, A. and E.V. Burnaev. (2018). Reinforcement learning in computer vision. In *Tenth International Conference on Machine Vision* (*ICMV 2017*), *10696*, pp. 458–464. SPIE.

Bittar, R., R. Bittar, A. Ptito, S.O. Dumoulin, M. Ptito, M. Ptito and J. Faubert. (1999). Activation of the remaining hemisphere following stimulation of the blind hemifield in hemi-spherectomized subjects. *NeuroImage*, *10*, 339–346.

Borisyuk, R., G. Borisyuk, C. Rallings and M. Thrasher. (2005). Forecasting the 2005 general election: A neural network approach. *The British Journal of Politics and Interna tional Relations*, *7*(2), 199–209.

Choudhary, R. and H.K. Gianey. (2017). Comprehensive review on supervised machine learning algorithms. In: *2017 International Conference on Machine Learning and Data Science* (*MLDS*), 37–43. IEEE.

de Oliveira Silva, A.S., F.S.Fonseca, M.V.S. Muniz, A.M.N. de Melo, W.G. Machado, M.A. de Santana and J. Carneiro. (2024). Enhancing ASD diagnosis with low-density EEG and machine learning. In: *Conference XXIX Congresso Brasileiro de Engenharia Biomedica* (*CBEB* 2024) até Ribeirão Preto.

Deb, K. (2001). *Multi-objective Optimization Using Evolutionary Algorithms*, pp. I–XIX, 1–497. Wiley, New York.

Dharshini, S.A.P., M.M. Gromiha and Y.H. Taguchi. (2019). Exploring the selective vulnerability in Alzheimer disease using tissue specific variant analysis. *Genomics*.

Domenico, M.D. (2017). Multilayer modeling and analysis of human brain networks. *Giga-Science*, *6*, 1–8.

Eberhart, R. (2007). *Computational Intelligence: Concepts to implementations*, pp. 496–496. ResearchGate.

El Naqa, I. and M.J. Murphy. (2015). *What is Machine Learning?* Springer.

Espinola, C.W., J.C. Gomes, J.M.S. Pereira and W.P. dos Santos. (2021a). Detection of major depressive disorder using vocal acoustic analysis and machine learning, an exploratory study. *Research on Biomedical Engineering*, *37*, 53–64.

Espinola, C.W., J.C. Gomes, J.M.S. Pereira and W.P. dos Santos. (2021b). Vocal acoustic analysis and machine learning for the identification of schizophrenia. *Research on Biomedical Engineering*, *37*, 33–46.

Favoretto, S., et al. (2016). *Máquinas de aprendizado extremo aplicadas a identificação de pessoas através de eletrocardiograma* (*ECG*). Master 's thesis, Universidade Tecnológica Federal do Paraná.

Freitag, C., M. Duan, P.G.P. Rosa, C. Francks, B. Bernhardt, G. Auzias, D. Murphy, K. Tammimies, S. Haar, D. Fair, S. Fisher, M.C. Postema, S. Durston, C. Ecker, M. Behrmann, E. Anagnostou, K. O'Hearn, K. Rubia, N. Jahanshad, M. Parellada, M. Jalbrzikowski, L. Gallagher, J. Buitelaar, P. Thompson, D. Floris, J. Janssen, E. Daly, Z. Sha, B. Luna, F.L.S. Duran, J. Fedor, J.A. King, S. Bolte, L. Hoekstra, B. Oranje, S. Ehrlich, A. Retico, G. Busatto, S. Calderoni, C. Deruelle, C.J. Molloy, R. Calvo, M.J. Taylor, C. Arango, F. Zhou, D. Glahn, J. Pariente, B. Franke, J. Fitzgerald, F. Muratori, D. van Rooij, J. McGrath, J. Neufeld, S. Medland, D.A. Shook, M. Tosetti, G. Wallace, K.L. Remnélius and L. Lázaro. (2021). Subtly altered topological asymmetry of brain structural covariance networks in autism spectrum disorder across 43 datasets from the enigma consortium. *Molecular Psychiatry*, *27*, 2114–2125.

Gomes, J.C., V.A. d.F. Barbosa, M.A. Santana, J. Bandeira, M.J.S. Valenc a, R.E. de Souza, A.M. Ismael and W.P. dos Santos. (2020). Ikonos: An intelligent tool to support diagnosis of COVID-19 by texture analysis of x-ray images. *Research on Biomedical Engineering*, 1–14.

Gomes, J.C., M.A. de Santana, A.I. Masood, C.L. de Lima and W.P. dos Santos. (2022). COVID-19's influence on cardiac function: A machine learning perspective on ECG analysis.

Gomes, J.C., V. Marques, C. de Brito, Y. Nascimento, G. Miranda, N. Córdula, C. Fragoso, A. Torcarte, M.A. Santana, G. Moreno, et al. (2023). Machine learning for detection and classification of motor imagery in electroencephalographic signals. In: *Biomedical Signal Processing*, pp. 149–171. CRC Press.

Gottlieb, J. and L. Snyder. (2010). Spatial and non-spatial functions of the parietal cortex. *Current Opinion in Neurobiology*, *20*, 731–740.

Gottwald, S. (2005). Mathematical fuzzy logic as a tool for the treatment of vague information. *Inf. Sci.*, *172*, 41–71.

Grossi, E. and M. Buscema. (2007). Introduction to artificial neural networks. *European Journal of Gastroenterology and Hepatology*, *19*(12), 1046–1054.

Hadders-Algra, M. (2018). Early human brain development: Starring the subplate. *Neuro science Biobehavioral Reviews*, *92*, 276–290.

Hahn, P. (2019). Artificial intelligence and machine learning. *Handchirurgie, Mikrochirurgie, Plastische Chirurgie: Organ der Deutschsprachigen Arbeitsgemeinschaft für Handchirurgie: Organ der Deutschsprachigen Arbeitsgemeinschaft für Mikrochirurgie der Peripheren Nerven und Gefäße: Organ der V...*, *51*(1), 62–67.

Haykin, S. (2001). Neural networks: Principles and practice. *Bookman*, *11*, 900.

Homan, R.W., J. Herman and P. Purdy. (1987). Cerebral location of international 10–20 system electrode placement. *Electroencephalography and Clinical Neurophysiology*, *66*(4), 376–382.

Jahedi, A., A.E. Abbott, R. Müller, M. Datko, I. Fishman, A. Nair and C. Keown. (2016). Patterns of atypical functional connectivity and behavioral links in autism differ between default, salience, and executive networks. *Cerebral Cortex*, *26* (10), 4034–4045.

Jefferies, E., K. Krieger-Redwood, B. Bernhardt, G. Hallam, J. Smallwood, I.D. Caso, J. Davey, T. Karapanagiotidis, C. Murphy and H. Edwards. (2016). Exploring the role of the posterior middle temporal gyrus in semantic cognition: Integration of anterior temporal lobe with executive processes. *Neuroimage*, *137*, 165–177.

Jhaveri, R., A. Revathi, K. Ramana, R. Raut and R.K. Dhanaraj. A review on machine learning strategies for real-world engineering applications. *Mobile Information Systems*, 2022.

Jiang, T., J.L. Gradus and A.J. Rosellini. (2020). Supervised machine learning: A brief primer. *Behavior Therapy*, *51*(5), 675–687.

Ju, H. and D. Bassett. (2020). Dynamic representations in networked neural systems. *Nature Neuroscience*, *23*, 908–917.

Krogh, A. (2008). What are artificial neural networks? *Nature Biotechnology*, *26*(2), 195–197.

LeCun, Y., L. Bottou, Y. Bengio and P. Haffner. (1998). Gradient-based learning applied to document recognition. *Proceedings of the IEEE*, *86*(11), 2278–2324.

LeCun, Y., Y. Bengio and G. Hinton. (2015). Deep learning. *Nature*, *521*(7553), 436–444.

Liu, J., Z. Cui, X. Liao, Z. Xu, X. Shou, M. Xia, Y. Xie and Y. He. (2021). Alterations in connectome dynamics in autism spectrum disorder: A harmonized mega- and meta-analysis study using the autism brain imaging data exchange dataset. *Biological Psychiatry*, *91*, 945–955.

Luo, L. (2021). Architectures of neuronal circuits. *Science*, *373*.

Mahajan, S. (2014). Reinforcement learning: A review from a machine learning perspective. *International Journal*, *4*(8).

Mastrogiuseppe, F., S. Ostojic, M. Beirán, A. Dubreuil and A. Valente. (2022). The role of population structure in computations through neural dynamics. *Nature Neuroscience*, *25*, 783–794.

McCulloch, W.S. and W. Pitts. (1943). A logical calculus of the ideas immanent in nervous activity. *The Bulletin of Mathematical Biophysics*, *5*, 115–133.

McLane, H.C., A.L. Berkowitz, B.N. Patenaude, E.D. McKenzie, E. Wolper, S. Wahlster, G. Fink and F.J. Mateen. (2015). Availability, accessibility, and affordability of neurodiagnostic tests in 37 countries. *Neurology*, *85*(18), 1614–1622.

Minsky, M. and S. Papert. (1969). An introduction to computational geometry. *Cambridge Tiass., HIT*, *479*(480), 104.

Mohammad-Rezazadeh, I., J. Frohlich, S. Loo and S. Jeste. (2016). Brain connectivity in autism spectrum disorder. *Current Opinion in Neurology*, *29* (2), 137–147.

Naydenov, K., A. Yordanova and V. Mancheva. (2022). Methodology for eeg and reference values of the software analysis. *Open Access Macedonian Journal of Medical Sciences*.

Niu, H., Q. Dong, U. and L. Cai. (2018). The development of functional network organization in early childhood and early adolescence: A resting-state first study. *Developmental Cognitive Neuroscience*, *30*, 223–235.

Nordahl, C., V.P. Reinhardt, A. Iosif, E. Ferrer, D. Amaral, S. Rogers, S. Ghetti, L.E. Libero, M. Solomon and B. Heath. (2020). Understanding hippocampal development in young children with autism spectrum disorder. *Journal of the American Academy of Child and Adolescent Psychiatry*.

Ojanguren, E.I. (2018). Computational intelligence. *Springer Theses*.

Palejwala, A.H., N. Dadario, I. Young, K. P. O'Connor, R.G. Briggs, A.K. Conner, D.L. O'Donoghue and M. Sughrue. (2021). Anatomy and white matter connections of the lingual gyrus and cuneus. *World Neurosurgery*.

Panikratova, Y.R., I. Kolykhalov, N. Cherkasov, I.S. Lebedeva, E. Abdullina, A.Y. Komarova, O. Bozhko and S.I. Gavrilova. (2-025). Functional connectivity within temporal brain regions and conversion to Alzheimer's disease in amnestic mild cognitive impairment. *Psychiatry* (*Moscow*) (*Psikhiatriya*).

Park, D., J. Griffiths, D. Mabbott, R. Noori, P. Frankland, J. Lefebvre and S. Bells. (2020). Activity-dependent myelination: A glial mechanism of oscillatory self-organization in large-scale brain networks. *Proceedings of the National Academy of Sciences*, *117*, 13227–13237.

Paszkiel, S. Data acquisition methods for human brain activity. *Analysis and Classification of EEG Signals for Brain–Computer Interfaces*, 2019.

Pereira, J.M., M.A. Santana, J.C. Gomes, V. A. de Freitas Barbosa, M.J.S. Valença, S.M.L. de Lima and W.P. dos Santos. (2021). Feature selection based on dialectics to support breast cancer diagnosis using thermographic images. *Research on Biomedical Engineering*, *37*, 485–506.

Roberts, T., J. Edgar, L. Blaskey and L. Cornew. (2012). Resting-state oscillatory activity in autism spectrum disorders. *Journal of Autism and Developmental Disorders*, *42*, 1884–1894.

Ruan, J., H. Luo, S. Liang, M. Lü, G. Chen, Z. Zheng, L. Ruan, X. Chen, D. Zhang, C. Li and M. Yao. (2024). Brain functional gradient and structure features in adolescent and adult autism spectrum disorders. *Human Brain Mapping*, *45*.

Sadeghi-Naini, A., F. Lu, S. Gandhi, E. Rakovitch, W. Tran, B. Curpen, M. Brackstone and N. Meti. (2020). Computational radiology in breast cancer screening and diagnosis using artificial intelligence. *Canadian Association of Radiologists Journal*, *72*, 98–108.

Santana, M.A., J.C. Gomes, A.S. Torcate, F.S. Fonseca, A. Suarez, G.M. Souza, G.M. Moreno and W.P. dos Santos. (2022). Emotion recognition from electroencephalographic and peripheral physiological signals using artificial intelligence with explicit features. In: *Biomedical Signal Processing*, pp. 172–197. CRC Press.

Shachmurove, Y., et al. (2002). *Applying Artificial Neural Networks to Business, Economics, and Finance*. Citeseer.

Shao, J., A.S. Persichetti, A. Martin and S. Gotts. (2024). A functional parcellation of the whole brain in high-functioning individuals with autism spectrum disorder reveals atypical patterns of network organization. *Molecular Psychiatry*, *30*, 1518–1528

Shirahige, L., B. Leimig, A. Baltar, A. Bezerra, C.V. F. de Brito, Y.S.O. do Nascimento, J.C. Gomes, W.-P. Teo, W.P. Dos Santos, M. Cairrão, et al. (2022). Classification of parkinson's disease motor phenotype: A machine learning approach. *Journal of Neural Transmission*, *129*(12), 1447–1461.

Silva, O., A.S.d. (2024). *Aplicação de aprendizado de máquina em sinais de EEG para o diagnóstico do transtorno do espectro autista*. Dissertação de mestrado, Universidade Federal de Pernambuco, Recife. URL https://repositorio.ufpe.br/handle/123456789/62786.

Singh, P. Supervised machine learning. *Learn PySpark: Build Python-Based Machine Learning and Deep Learning Models*, 117–159, 2019.

Souza, G.M.d. (2025). *Representação de sinais de EEG em imagens para o diagnóstico de Alzheimer: Uma abordagem baseada em deep learning e métodos de interpretabilidade*. Dissertação de mestrado, Universidade Federal de Pernambuco, Recife. Masters Dissertation.

Stuss, D. Functions of the frontal lobes: Relation to executive functions. *Journal of the International Neuropsychological Society*, *17*, 759–765, 2011.

Teplan, M., et al. (2002). Fundamentals of EEG measurement. *Measurement Science Review*, *2* (2), 1–11.

Theckedath, D. and R. Sedamkar. (2020). Detecting affect states using VGG 16, Res Net50 and SE-Res Net50 networks. *SN Computer Science*, *1*(2), 79.

Valko, N. and V. Osadchyi. (2020). Education individualization by means of artificial neural networks. *E3S Web of Conferences*, 166(4), 2021. ResearchGate.

Vaziri-Pashkam, M. and Y. Xu. (2017). Goal-directed visual processing differentially impacts human ventral and dorsal visual representations. *The Journal of Neuroscience*, *37*, 8767–8782.

Vecchio, F., F. Miraglia, C. Marra, D. Quaranta, M. Vita, P. Bramanti and P. Rossini. (2014). Human brain networks in cognitive decline: A graph theoretical analysis of cortical connectivity from EEG data. *Journal of Alzheimer's Disease: JAD*, *41*(1), 113–127.

Vermeulen, A.F. (2020). Unsupervised learning: Using unlabeled data. *Industrial Machine Learning: Using Artificial Intelligence as a Transformational Disruptor*, pp. 181–206.

Wani, P. (2024). From sound to meaning: Navigating Wernicke's area in language processing. *Cureus*, *16*.

Zapirain, B.G., I.D.L.T. Díez and S.G. Alonso. (2019). Predictive, personalized, preventive, and participatory (4p) medicine applied to telemedicine and e-health in the literature. *Journal of Medical Systems*, *43*, 1–10.

Zarifi, T., C.-C. Peng and M.H. Zarifi. (2011). Low-power amplifier for *in vivo* eeg signal recording. In: *2011 1st Middle East Conference on Biomedical Engineering*, pp. 19–22, IEEE.

2 Autism Spectrum Disorder
Overview and the Historical Path of Diagnosis

Karla Amorim Sancho[1*], Fabiano Tonaco Borges[1]

The chapter presents an overview and the historical path of Autism Spectrum Disorder diagnosis. It begins with a discussion of the challenges in early identification. It highlights core features: difficulties in social communication, repetitive behaviors, and restricted interests. The analysis covers global and regional prevalence of ASD. It addresses variations in diagnostic criteria and barriers to healthcare access. The text examines the evolution of the autism concept. It starts with Leo Kanner's initial description in 1943. It moves to Hans Asperger's recognition in the 1980s. It culminates with the modern definition of the "autism spectrum" in the DSM-5. The chapter underscores the influence of historical, social, and scientific factors on diagnostic practices. It also describes advances in knowledge about the genetic and environmental bases of the disorder. It concludes by stressing the importance of multidisciplinary approaches in diagnosis and treatment. It calls for inclusive public policies. These policies provide lifelong support for individuals with ASD, encourage social integration, and improve quality of life.

1. Introduction

In this chapter, we propose a comprehensive analysis of Autism Spectrum Disorder (ASD). We aim to offer an overview of this condition. It affects neurodevelopment[#] and significantly influences communication, social interaction, and behavior. Over recent decades, our understanding of autism has changed in many ways. These changes reveal shifts in scientific, diagnostic, and social approaches.

1 Universidade Federal de Pernambuco, Brazil.
* Corresponding author: karla.amorims@ufpe.br.

Masculine noun. [Medicine] Development of the nervous system. This process covers motor skills, manipulation, sensory abilities, communication and language, behaviors, cognitive skills, affect, and emotions (for example, child neurodevelopment). "Neurodevelopment." In: Dicionário Priberam da Língua Portuguesa [online], 2008–2024. Available at: <https://dicionario.priberam.org/neurodesenvolvimento>. Access on: 26 Oct. 2024.

DOI: 10.1201/9781003531418-2

The chapter also traces a detailed historical journey. It starts with Leo Kanner's and Hans Asperger's earliest clinical descriptions. It moves to the current diagnostic criteria outlined in the DSM-5. We address the complexity of the autism spectrum and the historical development of its diagnosis. We note how experts first viewed autism as a rare and isolated disorder. We now regard it as a multifaceted condition that involves a broad range of characteristics and levels of severity. This perspective underscores the importance of historical and contextual awareness. It helps us understand advances and challenges in identifying and supporting people with ASD.

2. Overview

ASD is a neurodevelopmental condition. Its signs can emerge within the first 12 months of life (Maestro et al., 2005). In some cases, symptoms appear as early as the first 6 months (Tanner et al., 2020; Sarret et al., 2015). Clinicians often diagnose ASD around 24 months of age (Zwaigenbaum et al., 2016). However, the average age at diagnosis ranges from 2.7 to 7.2 years (Loubersac et al., 2021).

This disorder causes significant challenges in communication and social interaction. It also involves repetitive behaviors and restricted interests. Individuals with ASD often show heightened sensory sensitivity. They may respond atypically to visual, auditory, or tactile stimuli (Napolitano et al., 2022). Symptom variability creates a unique experience of autism for each person. As a result, diagnosis and intervention demand a highly personalized approach.

The prevalence and incidence of ASD cases vary by source. These variations reflect the different methods that researchers use for data collection and analysis. Globally, an estimated 98 in every 10,000 individuals receive an ASD diagnosis (Wang et al., 2022).

Recent studies show a rise in Autism Spectrum Disorder prevalence in the United States. In 2016, the estimated prevalence among children aged 3–17 years reached 2.50% (Xu et al., 2019). It rose to 2.85% in 2019–2020 (Li et al., 2022). Among 8-year-olds, prevalence stood at 18.5 per 1,000 (1 in 54) in 2016 (Maenner et al., 2020). Prevalence varies across states. It ranges from 1.54% in Texas to 4.88% in Florida (Xu et al., 2019).

ASD appears 4.3 times more often in boys than in girls (Maenner et al., 2020). About 70% of children with ASD receive treatment. Another 29.5% receive neither behavioral nor medication interventions (Xu et al., 2019). Racial and ethnic disparities remain in early evaluation and diagnosis. Black and Hispanic children encounter more delays in identification and intervention (Maenner et al., 2020).

In Brazil, one in every 59 children receives this diagnosis, according to some studies (Molini et al., 2021). These data show that ASD appears in many cultures and social classes. However, De Oliveira Silva (2024) warns that current estimates may not capture the true prevalence. This gap becomes more pronounced in regions with limited access to specialized healthcare services, where diagnostic challenges intensify.

According to the same author, underreporting of ASD increases because families often lack awareness of early autism signs. Professionals in healthcare, education, and daily childcare also lack sufficient information. This shortfall in knowledge complicates early detection and leads to delays in interventions. Timely interventions can significantly improve prognoses and quality of life for children with ASD.

Currently, specialists rely on a predominantly clinical approach to diagnosed ASD. They base this process on behavioral evaluations. Multidisciplinary teams—comprising psychiatrists, clinical psychologists, and neuropsychologists—combine direct observations with standardized questionnaires (Heinsfeld et al., 2018; Khodatars et al., 2021). This strategy ensures accuracy and depth in the diagnostic process.

However, in Brazil, specialists are often unavailable, especially in under-resourced regions. This limitation makes it hard to implement a broad clinical approach. Early ASD diagnosis encounters major obstacles. The shortage of specialized professionals in many parts of the country lengthens evaluation and diagnosis. This delay blocks timely interventions. It may also worsen secondary issues, such as academic problems, social isolation, and increased anxiety or depression (Bajestani et al., 2019). Early identification and intervention are crucial. They give children with ASD the best possible prognosis.

Symptom diversity adds more challenges. ASD spans deficits in communication and repetitive behavioral patterns. This wide range often causes misunderstandings or incorrect diagnoses. Some may see communication difficulties as isolated speech issues. Others may view repetitive behaviors as harmless quirks. These misinterpretations prevent accurate or prompt diagnosis. They deny children and families the therapeutic interventions that prove most effective when introduced early (Hus et al., 2021).

The exact etiology of Autism Spectrum Disorder remains unclear. Researchers conduct intensive studies to explore the multiple dimensions of this complex neurodevelopmental disorder. Substantial evidence highlights the significant role of genetic factors in the condition. Yet, no single gene or mutation explains ASD. Studies indicate a heritable predisposition, but the specific contribution of individual genes to the disorder remains unknown and calls for further exploration (Torre-Ubieta et al., 2016; Yoon et al., 2020).

Environmental factors also play a relevant part in ASD. Complications during pregnancy, early exposure to certain substances or environmental conditions, and other related events increase the risk of its onset. Scientists continue to investigate these scenarios to clarify how genetic and environmental factors interact. This line of inquiry draws strong interest and drives ongoing research (Yoon et al., 2020).

The absence of a single, clearly defined cause for ASD reflects its complexity. This fact suggests that its etiology likely results from an interaction of multiple factors. This scenario underscores the need for a multifaceted, integrated approach to fully comprehend and address the disorder. Such an approach acknowledges the wide range of influences that shape its development and manifestation (Parellada et al., 2014).

Clinicians use the *DSM-5* (*Diagnostic and Statistical Manual of Mental Disorders*, Fifth Edition) criteria to diagnose ASD. The American Psychiatric Association published the *DSM-5* in 2013. It combined multiple conditions previously listed separately—such as classic autism, Asperger syndrome, and pervasive developmental disorder not otherwise specified—under the single term "Autism Spectrum Disorder" (Association et al., 2002).

This change simplified diagnostic criteria. It introduced significant challenges in standardizing the diagnosis. This issue grows more complex in public health systems with limited resources. According to the *DSM-5*, ASD diagnostic criteria include persistent deficits in socioemotional reciprocity, nonverbal communication challenges, and social interaction difficulties. They also involve stereotypic behaviors and restricted interests. The disorder covers a broad range of atypical sensory responses, from hypersensitivity to hyposensitivity to sensory stimuli. These features illustrate the complexity and diversity of ASD.

The *DSM-5* criteria aim to ensure accurate, standardized evaluations. They consider the complexity and variability of ASD symptoms. Clinicians use these criteria together with detailed clinical assessments. They pursue a comprehensive and personalized diagnostic approach. This strategy identifies each individual's specific needs and addresses them. It promotes more effective, targeted interventions (Association et al., 2002).

According to De Oliveira Silva (2024), the classification of Autism Spectrum Disorder relies on the level of support needed. It splits into three distinct categories. At Level 1, individuals face difficulties in social communication skills and daily tasks. They still maintain a significant degree of independence. They benefit from support that targets social and organizational skills, with specific interventions that foster social integration and daily functioning.

At Level 2, deficits grow more pronounced. Individuals show significant difficulties in communication and behavior. They need substantial support in many areas of daily life. Interventions focus on addressing communication challenges and aiding adaptation to daily routines and demands. At Level 3, deficits become severe. They strongly affect communication and involve highly restrictive, repetitive behaviors. Individuals at this level rely on continuous assistance to complete basic activities and maintain well-being. They need intensive, continuous support to uphold functionality and quality of life. This categorization allows a tailored approach for each person's specific needs, as Gardner et al. (2018) describe.

After we understand the main features of ASD and the complexity involved in its identification, we must explore how this diagnosis changed over time. The historical path of ASD diagnosis reveals changes in scientific and clinical approaches. It also reflects cultural, social, and technological influences that shape how we currently understand and categorize this condition. This analysis places advances in autism identification in context. It highlights the challenges that were overcome and those that remain. It also emphasizes the importance of a historical perspective for understanding the foundations of modern diagnosis.

3. Historical Path of Diagnosis

Clinical diagnosis stands as a key medical practice. Social, cultural, and ideological factors shape its history. They echo the historical circumstances of its development. According to Sancho et al. (2019), diagnosis is not only an objective medical category. It is also a discourse in constant evolution, guided by ideological disputes and discursive memories[#] that shifts its meaning over time. By examining the historical path of diagnosis, we see how changes in clinical practice and social relations influenced the formation of ASD diagnosis. This section addresses those historical changes, highlighting milestones and debates that established the diagnostic framework we recognize today.

Fadda (2020) notes that people described autism-compatible behaviors in many cultures throughout history. However, Leo Kanner only formalized the diagnosis in 1943 when he examined 11 children who showed similar behavioral symptoms. Among them, Donald Gray Triplett stood out. Experts consider him "case number one" of autism, given his striking introspection

[#] One defines discursive formation in relation to ideological formation: "Ideological formations [...] necessarily include, as one of their components, one or more interrelated discursive formations. They determine what a person can and must say (expressed as a harangue, sermon, pamphlet, exposition, program, etc.) from a given position at a specific point in time" (Haroche et al., 1971, p. 32).

and social isolation. The etymological origin of the term 'autism' reinforces this feature. It alludes to a focus on the "self," emphasizing individuality and detachment from the outside world (Haney, 2015, p. 90).

According to Fadda (2020), experts officially recognized autism as a category separate from schizophrenia in 1980. This milestone represented a significant advance with the release of the DSM-III by the American Psychiatric Association (American Psychiatric Association, 1989). Initially, specialists viewed autism as a rare condition that affected about 4 in every 10,000 children born in the United States, as Frith (1989) observed. However, understanding of the disorder evolved. Baio et al. (2018) estimate a current prevalence of 1 in every 59 children in the US. This rise reflects broader diagnostic criteria and increased autism awareness, which allowed experts to detect cases that previously went unnoticed.

Fadda (2020) states that developmental impairments from ASD usually appear in the first months of life. They strongly affect how the child sees the self, others, and the environment. As a result, these children often avoid spontaneous social contact. They rarely make direct eye contact with those who approach them. When they do, they look sideways and only for brief moments. They also show language differences. Even with strong verbal articulation, their speech often seems distinctive. In some cases, it has a monotone intonation. Their interests are narrow and repetitive. This pattern complicates their participation in shared activities and common interests (Asperger, 1991/1944; Kanner, 1943; Jerusalinsky, 2015; Muratori, 2014).

The *DSM-5* (American Psychiatric Association, 2014) currently defines autism as a neurodevelopmental disorder that covers a wide range of symptoms. This scope justifies the use of the term 'spectrum'. Clinicians diagnose ASD by combining retrospective information with current observations. They also consider whether a person has learned to hide or compensate for symptoms over time. However, autism persists throughout life. Symptoms may vary in intensity, but it does not allow a person to "leave the spectrum", unlike older perspectives in the DSM-IV. Early interventions can improve symptoms, but the diagnosis remains for life.

Although experts view autism as a lifelong condition, scientific literature focuses mostly on the early years. This emphasis occurs because early therapeutic interventions can significantly improve clinical symptoms (Landa, 2018). However, this focus neglects many adults with the same diagnosis. They often face serious obstacles when they try to participate in society. Medication remains the only treatment option for these individuals. This limitation likely stems from a shortage of specific knowledge and professional competence that could open the way for more diverse and effective therapeutic approaches (Brugha et al., 2015).

A narrow perspective and restricted focus on early interventions reveal gaps in lifelong care. They also reflect historical challenges related to the diagnosis and approach to autism. An exploration of the historical evolution of the concept and diagnosis of autism clarifies how these gaps emerged. The historical context shows how social, cultural, and scientific factors shaped our current view of the disorder. It traces the journey from the earliest clinical descriptions to contemporary approaches. It highlights progress and persistent barriers in recognizing and supporting individuals with autism.

4. History of the Concept of Autism

The autism spectrum covers a broad range of human developmental disorders. These disorders show deviations that appear in the earliest years of life. The clinical expression of this spectrum includes severe cases, such as infantile autism described by Kanner (1943), and milder cases, such as Asperger syndrome identified by Asperger (1944/1991). Different levels of affective contact restriction and behavioral rigidity interconnect these extremes. Their intensity varies among individuals.

The concept of autism has gone through many shifts and reinterpretations over time. It absorbs sociohistorical changes that reflect the consensus and disagreements formed over more than a century of progress in Psychiatry and Psychopathology. Using the word 'autism' in retrospective analyses may cause misunderstandings. The meaning attached to the term changed considerably throughout this condition's history. Diagnoses also faced constant revision, in line with the evolution of scientific concepts and approaches.

Fadda (2020) presents a summary of this historical path. According to the author, Emil Kraepelin's first edition of the *Compendium of Psychiatry* (*Compendium der Psychiatrie*) appeared in Germany in 1883. It marked an important milestone in the systematization of psychiatric knowledge. Between 1884 and 1886, Edmund Husserl explored intentionality and psychic processes under Franz Brentano's guidance, which enriched the emerging field of Psychology. Sigmund Freud had also studied with Brentano for almost two years at the University of Vienna, a period that influenced Psychoanalysis in its early stages.

In the Compendium—later renamed Treatise—Emil Kraepelin revised and refined the concept of "dementia praecox". He defined it as a progressive breakdown in affective, intellectual, and volitional domains. In the sixth edition, published in 1899, he established it as a well-defined nosographic entity (Pessotti, 2007). In 1906, Sancte de Sanctis observed 25 children, aged 6, 7, and 10, whose symptoms matched Kraepelin's description. He called it "very early dementia". In 1908, Heller studied children between three and four years of age who showed mannerisms and stereotyped speech. He named that condition "infantile dementia" (Marfinati and Abrão, 2014; Wolff, 2004).

Eugen Bleuler, a Swiss psychiatrist, introduced the term 'autism' in 1911. He linked it to schizophrenia as a feature that suggested detachment from the external world. However, in 1943, Leo Kanner offered the first detailed clinical description of children with what he called "infantile autism". He depicted these children as having an innate inability to form normal affective ties with others and an intense focus on repetitive activities.

During that period, Eugen Bleuler wished to diverge from Emil Kraepelin's ideas. Kraepelin viewed mental disorders as results of purely organic causes. Bleuler, on the other hand, drew closer to psychoanalysis, an emerging clinical approach that explained schizophrenia based on psychological factors (Reis, 2000). In that context, Bleuler saw autism as an effect of schizophrenia. He described it as a "predominance of interior life and active detachment from the external world" (Tatossian, 2006, p. 57). This concept resembled Freud's idea of autoerotism (Lara, 2012; Oliveira, 2000).

Around the same time, while Bleuler linked autism to schizophrenia, Karl Jaspers published the influential book *General Psychopathology* in Germany in 1913. In that work, Jaspers employed Edmund Husserl's phenomenological method. He aimed to accomplish two main goals. First, he intended to find a broad principle that would explain various manifestations of human experiences by addressing fundamental concepts and principles. Second, he proposed a scientific approach to validate 'subjective' symptoms, which earlier science had not measured with traditional methods (Moreira, 2011).

Fadda (2020) observes significant worldwide transformations then, especially in mental health and the understanding of childhood. In Switzerland, in 1921, Herman Rorschach published *Psychodiagnostics*, based on how people responded to inkblot cards. In 1922, Eugene Minkowski and Ludwig Binswanger—both former Bleuler assistants—presented their work at the Swiss Society of Psychiatry in Zurich. They used phenomenological philosophy to address psychiatric clinical practice (Moreira, 2011). The following year, Jean Piaget published *The Language and Thought of the Child*, his first book devoted to childhood studies. Meanwhile, in Germany, between 1922 and 1923, Melanie Klein applied psychoanalysis to children. In the United States, the National Committee for Mental Hygiene financed clinics focused on child care, including Bellevue Hospital in New York. That facility opened a dedicated ward for Child Psychiatry (American Academy of Child & Adolescent Psychiatry, s.d.; Whonamedit, s.d.; Moreira, 2011).

Child psychiatry took shape as a distinct field. Its aim went beyond labeling childhood psychoses or organic-based delays (Marfinati and Abrão,

2014). In this context, Leo Kanner moved to the United States in 1924 to seek new opportunities. At that time, no formal Pediatric Psychiatry courses existed. Kanner taught himself while working as an assistant physician at the State Hospital in Yankton, South Dakota. In 1930, Johns Hopkins University asked him to create the first child psychiatry service in the United States (American Academy of Child & Adolescent Psychiatry, s.d.; Johns Hopkins Children's Center, 2017; Whonamedit, s.d.). He then conducted a series of analyses on childhood phenomena, publishing most of his work in the *Journal of Pediatrics* (Kanner, 1933, 1934, 1937a, 1937b, 1938a, 1938b, 1939, 1940, 1943, 1944; Conn and Kanner, 1940).

During this same period, J. L. Despert described children with traits labeled "infantile schizophrenia". Experts now recognize those traits as features of the autism spectrum (Marfinati and Abrão, 2014). Carl Rogers published his first book in 1939, titled *The Clinical Treatment of the Problem Child*. Researchers began developing various child scales, including Arnold Gesell's. In 1943, Kanner used that scale to observe a lack of anticipatory behavior in children under his clinical care.

Fadda (2020) notes that global interest in child development was rising. In 1938, parents with high educational backgrounds started contacting Leo Kanner. They described children who showed unusual or challenging behaviors. His extensive clinical experience led to the first formal characterization and conceptualization of infantile autism in 1943.

What propelled Kanner to global recognition as a pioneer in autism studies, even though other professionals had already identified and described similar characteristics? According to Grinker (2010) and Oliveira (2000), his recognition came from a mix of historical and political factors.

In the United States, Kanner acted as a trailblazer in many respects. He was the first in the Americas to publish a book titled *Child Psychiatry* in 1935, establishing this field as an independent medical discipline. He was also the first physician officially recognized as a child psychiatrist (Johns Hopkins Children's Center, 2017). He stood out by consistently publishing numerous articles on child and adolescent mental health. This prolific output strengthened his authority on the subject.

During the 1940s, Hans Asperger described children who showed behaviors similar to those Kanner observed. These children had linguistic and cognitive development within expected ranges. They showed social and behavioral difficulties but had normal intellectual capacities. Asperger used the term "autistic psychopathy" for these presentations. However, his work stayed largely unknown outside Europe until the 1980s, when the psychologist Lorna Wing revisited Asperger's research and introduced the term "Asperger Syndrome".

During and after World War II, political and ideological barriers limited the access of American and British psychiatrists to Central European research. The postwar era brought an increase in psychiatric admissions and advances in mental health knowledge. Professionals published the *DSM-I* in 1952 and introduced chlorpromazine as the first antipsychotic. At that time, autism emerged as a distinct entity. Leo Kanner gained recognition for his pioneering work, although experts still debated organic versus psychological causes of the disorder.

In the 1970s, researchers such as Israel Kolvin and Michael Rutter expanded the distinction between autism and schizophrenia. They highlighted genetic factors and refined diagnostic criteria. The *DSM-III*, in 1980, classified autism as a pervasive developmental disorder. This decision established autism as an independent category. During the same period, Lorna Wing revisited Hans Asperger's research on children with autistic traits, which had remained obscure. She introduced Asperger syndrome to the academic setting. Kanner and Asperger approached autism with different priorities. Kanner emphasized precise diagnostic boundaries, while Asperger focused on educational aspects.

In 2013, the *DSM-5* consolidated the concept of the autism spectrum. The ICD-11 adopted this perspective in 2018. This modern view integrates contributions from many researchers, including Kanner and Asperger. It underlines the clinical and diagnostic evolution of autism while recognizing its complexity and diverse manifestations (Grinker, 2010; Oliveira, 2000).

5. Impact of Early Diagnosis and Interventions

Experts see early diagnosis of ASD as a key factor for successful intervention. Therapeutic measures in the early years bring significant improvements in the behavioral and social symptoms of children with ASD. Behavioral therapy and speech therapy stand out as common and effective approaches to enhance their communication and interaction skills.

Despite the scientific focus on autism in children, many autistic adults still face considerable challenges, especially with social inclusion. Clinicians rarely address adult diagnosis, and these individuals often rely on medication as their only treatment option. Many adults with ASD struggle to integrate into society, and they lack specialized support tailored to their needs.

The neurodiversity movement has gained momentum in recent years. It promotes a broader, more inclusive understanding of autism as a natural variation of the human condition, not merely a pathology. This perspective values unique traits and "islands of excellence" that many autistic people display. It stresses that society must adapt to include them, rather than expecting them to conform to established social norms.

6. The Future of Autism: Perspectives and Challenges

ASD affects people in varied and complex ways. Research has progressed, but many challenges persist, especially for adults with autism. Early diagnosis and interventions matter. Yet professionals must expand their focus and provide ongoing support throughout an autistic person's life.

Scientists in genetics and neuroscience continue to investigate autism's underlying causes. They study genetic and environmental factors that contribute to the condition. A multidisciplinary diagnostic approach is crucial. Psychiatrists, psychologists, occupational therapists, and other health professionals coordinate efforts to deliver personalized treatment.

De Oliveira Silva (2024) emphasizes the need for public policies that raise awareness at all levels of society. These policies must include continuous training for health professionals, educators, and caregivers. Early interventions can decisively change the outcomes for children and foster their development and social inclusion.

The neurodiversity movement poses essential questions about how society views autism. It avoids labeling differences as pathologies. It sees autism as part of the natural range of human experience. Inclusion and individualized support remain central goals.

References

American Academy of Child and Adolescent Psychiatry. (sem data). *AACAP History*. Disponível em: <https://www.aacap.org/AACAP/About_AACAP/AACAP_History.aspx.

Whonamedit>. (sem data). Acesso em: 05 dez 2019.

Asperger, H. (1991). "Autistic psychopathy" in childhood. Em U. Frith (Trad.), *Autism and Asperger Syndrome*, pp. 37–92. Cambridge, Reino Unido: Cambridge University. (Original Publicado em 1944).

Associação Americana de Psiquiatria. (2014). *Manual diagnóstico e estatístico de transtornos mentais: DSM-5*. (M.I.C. Nascimento, Trad.) (5a Ed.). Porto Alegre, RS: Artmed. (Original Publicado em 2013).

Association, A.P., et al. (2002). *Manual diagnóstico e estatístico de transtornos mentais*. [S.l.: s.n.].

Baio, J., Wiggins, L., Christensen, D.L., et al. (2018). Prevalence of Autism Spectrum Disorder Among Children Aged 8 Years: Autism and Developmental Disabilities Monitoring Network, 11 Sites, United States, 2014. *MMWR Surveillance Summaries*, *67*(6), 1–23. doi:10.15585/mmwr.ss6706a1.

Bajestani, G.S., Behrooz, M., Khani, A.G., Nouri, M. and Mollaei, A. (2019). Diagnosis of autism spectrum disorder based on complex network features. *Computer Methods and Programs in Biomedicine*, *177*, 277–283.

Brugha, T.S., Doos, L., Tempier, A., Einfeld, S. and Howlin, P. (2015). Outcome measures in intervention trials for adults with Autism spectrum disorders; A systematic review of assessments of core Autism features and associated emotional and behavioural problems. *International Journal of Methods in Psychiatric Research*, *24*(2), 99–115. doi:10.1002/mpr.1466.

Conn, J.H., and Kanner, L. (1940). Spontaneous erections in early childhood. *The Journal of Pediatrics*, *16*(3), 337–340. doi:10.1016/S0022-3476(40)80153-4.

De Oliveira Silva, A.S. (2024). *Aplicação de Aprendizado de Máquina em Sinais de EEG para o Diagnóstico do Transtorno do Espectro Autista*. Dissertação (mestrado), Programa de Pós-Graduação em Engenharia Biomédica da Universidade Federal de Pernambuco.

Fadda, G.M. (2020). *A experiência vivida por pessoas diagnosticadas como autistas, a partir de encontros dialógicos*. 200f. Tese (Doutorado em Psicologia)–Pontifícia Universidade Católica de Campinas, Centro de Ciências da Vida, Programa de Pós-Graduação em Psicologia, Campinas, 2020.

Frith, U. (1989). *Autism: Explain the Enigma*. Oxford, Inglaterra: Basil Blackwell.

Gardner, L.M., Campbell, J.M., Keisling, B. and Murphy, L. (2018). Correlates of DSM-5 autism spectrum disorder levels of support ratings in a clinical sample. *Journal of Autism and Developmental Disorders*, *48*(10), 3513–3523.

Grinker, R.R. (2010). *Autismo: Um mundo obscuro e conturbado* (C. Pinheiro, Trad.). São Paulo: Larousse do Brasil.

Haney, K. (2015). Verso uma fenomenologia dell'autismo. Em A. Ales Bello, G. Basti & A.M. Pezzella (Eds.). *Comunicazione Interativa: Intersoggetività, comunicazione, educazione*, pp. 87–117. Cidade do Vaticano. Itália: Universidade Lateranense.

Haroche, C., Henry, P. and Pêcheux, M. (1971). La sémantique et la coupure saussurienne: Langue, langage, discours. *Langages*, *24*, 93–106.

Heinsfeld, A.S., Franco, A.R., Craddock, R.C., Buchweitz, A., and Meneguzzi, F. (2018). Identification of autism spectrum disorder using deep learning and the abide dataset. *NeuroImage: Clinical*, *17*, 16–23.

Hus, Y. and Segal, O. (2021). Challenges surrounding the diagnosis of autism in children. *Neuropsychiatric Disease and Treatment*, *17*, 3509–3529.

Jerusalinsky, A. (Org.). (2015). *Dossiê Autismo*. São Paulo: Instituto Langage.

Johns Hopkins Children's Center. (2017). Founding of Child and Adolescent Psychiatry at Hopkins. Em Fellowship Program Prospectus 2017–2018. Acesso em: <https://www.hopkinsmedicine.org/psychiatry/specialty_areas/child_adolescent/child_educa tion/prospectus_child_2017.pdf>. Acesso em: 05 dez 2019.

Kanner, Leo. (2019). Disponível em: <http://www.whonamedit.com/doctor.cfm/2879.html>. Acesso em: 05 dez

Kanner, L. (1933). The significance of a pluralistic attitude in the study of human behavior. *The Journal of Abnormal and Social Psychology*, *28*(1), 30–41. doi:10.1037/h0072883.

Kanner, L. (1934). The occurrence of cataleptic phenomena in children. *The Journal of Pediatrics*, *5*(3), 330–340. doi:10.1016/S0022-3476(34)80052-2.

Kanner, L. (1937a). The invalid reaction in children. *The Journal of Pediatrics*, *11*(3), 341–355. doi:10.1016/S0022-3476(37)80021-9.

Kanner, L. (1937b). The development and present status of psychiatry in pediatrics. *The Journal of Pediatrics*, *11*(3), 418–435. doi:10.1016/S0022-3476(37)80027-X.

Kanner, L. (1938a). Some pediatric problems of behavior in infancy and early childhood. *The Journal of Pediatrics*, *13*(3), 417–433. doi:10.1016/S0022-3476(38)80150-5.

Kanner, L. (1938b). The Paediatric-Psychiatric Alliance. *Can. Med. Assoc. J.*, *38*(1), 71–74.

Kanner, L. (1939). Infantile sexuality. *The Journal of Pediatrics*, *15*(4), 583–608. doi:10.1016/S0022-3476(39)80018-X.

Kanner, L. (1940). Play investigation and play treatment of children's behavior disorders. *The Journal of Pediatrics*, *17*(4), 533–546. doi:10.1016/S0022-3476(40)80108-X.

Kanner, L. (1943). Autistic disturbances of affective contact. *Nervous Child*, 2, 217–250.

Kanner, L. (1944). Early Infantile Autism. *The Journal of Pediatrics*, *25*(3), 211–217. doi:10.1016/S0022-3476(44)80156-1.

Khodatars, M., Shoeibi, A., Sadeghi, D., Ghaasemi, N., Jafari, M., Moridian, P., Khadem, A., Alizadehsani, R., Zare, A. and Kong, Y. (2021). Deep learning for neuroimaging-based diagnosis and rehabilitation of autism spectrum disorder: A review. *Computers in Biology and Medicine*, *139*, 104949.

Landa, R.J. (2018). Efficacy of early interventions for infants and young children with, and at risk for, autism spectrum disorders. *International Review of Psychiatry*, *30*(1), 25–39. doi:10.1080/09540261.2018.1432574.

Lara, J.G. (2012). El autismo: Historia y clasificaciones. *Salud Mental*, *35*(3), 257–261.

Li, Q., Li, Y., Liu, B., Chen, Q., Xing, X., Xu, G. and Yang, W. (2022, Sep.). Prevalence of Autism Spectrum Disorder Among Children and Adolescents in the United States from 2019 to 2020. *JAMA Pediatr.*, *176*(9), 943–945. doi: 10.1001/jamapediatrics.2022.1846. PMID: 35789247; PMCID: PMC9257681.

Loubersac, J., Michelon, C., Ferrando, L., Picot, M. and Baghdadli, A. (2021). Predictors of an earlier diagnosis of autism spectrum disorder in children and adolescents: A systematic review (1987–2017). *European Child and Adolescent Psychiatry*, *32*, 375–393.

Maenner, M.J., Shaw, K.A., Baio, J., et al. (2016). Prevalence of Autism Spectrum Disorder Among Children Aged 8 Years: Autism and Developmental Disabilities Monitoring Network, 11 Sites, United States. *MMWR Surveill Summ 2020*; *69* (No. SS-4),1–12. doi: http://dx.doi.org/10.15585/mmwr.ss6904a1.

Maestro, S., Muratori, F., Cesari, A., Cavallaro, M., Paziente, A., Pecini, C., Grassi, C., Manfredi, A., and Sommario, C. (2005). Course of autism signs in the first year of life. *Psychopathology*, *38*, 26–31.

Marfinati, A. and Abrão, J.L. (2014). Um percurso pela psiquiatria infantil: Dos antecedentes históricos à origem do conceito de autismo. *Estilos da Clínica*, *19*(2), 244–262. doi:10.11606/issn.1981-1624.v19i2p244-262.

Molini-Avejonas, D. and Mandaj, V. (2021). Psychosocial care network for children with autism spectrum disorder in Brazil. *European Psychiatry*, *64*, S218–S218.

Moreira, V. (2011). A contribuição de Jaspers, Binswanger, Boss e Tatossian para a psicopatologia fenomenológica. *Revista da Abordagem Gestáltica*, *17*(2), 172–184.

Muratori, F. (2014). *O diagnóstico precoce no autismo: Guia prático para pediatras* (C. C. de Siervi & D.B. Wanderley, Trads.). Salvador, BA: Núcleo Interdisciplinar de Intervenção Precoce da Bahia.

Napolitano, A., Schiavi, S., Rosa, P.L., Rossi-Espagnet, M.C., Petrillo, S., Bottino, F., Tagliente, E., Longo, D., Lupi, E., Casula, L., Valeri, G., Piemonte, F., Trezza, V., and Vicari, S. (2022). Sex differences in autism spectrum disorder: Diagnostic, neurobiological, and behavioral features. *Frontiers in Psychiatry*, *13*.

Oliveira, L.E.P. de. (2000). Jeremias, criança, luta contra o autismo, a esquizofrenia e a paranóia. *Revista Latinoamericana de Psicopatologia Fundamental*, *3*(3), 73–102. doi:10.1590/1415-47142000003006.

Parellada, M., Penzol, M., Pina, L., Moreno, C., González-Vioque, E., Zalsman, G. and Arango, C. (2014). The neurobiology of autism spectrum disorders. *European Psychiatry*, *29*, 11–19.

Pessotti, I. (2007). Demência, dementia praecox, esquizofrenia. *O Que Nos Faz Pensar*, *16*(22), 113–143.

Reis, F.D. dos. (2000). Da demência precoce à esquizofrenia. *Psicologia*, *14*(1), 11–24. Disponível em: <http://www.scielo.mec.pt/scielo.php?script=sci_arttext&pid=S0874-20492000000100001&lng=pt&tlng=pt>. Acesso em: : 05 dez 2019.

Sancho, K.A., Pfeiffer, C.R.C. and Corrêa, C.R.S. (2019). Medicalização, diagnóstico clínico e queixa-conduta: Redes de significação em jogo. *Interface-Comunicação, Saúde, Educação*, *23*, e170633.

Sarrett, J.C. and Rommelfanger, K. (2015). Commentary: Attention to eyes is present but in decline in 2–6-month-old infants later diagnosed with autism. *Frontiers in Public Health*, *3*.

Tanner, A. and Dounavi, K. (2020). The emergence of autism symptoms prior to 18 months of age: A systematic literature review. *Journal of Autism and Developmental Disorders*, *51*, 973–993.

Tatossian, A. (2006). *Fenomenologia das psicoses*. São Paulo: Escuta.

Torre-Ubieta, L., Won, H., Stein, J. and Geschwind, D. (2016). Advancing the understanding of autism disease mechanisms through genetics. *Nature Medicine*, *22*, 345–361.

Wang, J., Ma, B., Wang, J., Zhang, Z. and Chen, Q. (2022). Global prevalence of autism spectrum disorder and its gastrointestinal symptoms: A systematic review and meta-analysis. *Frontiers in Psychiatry*, *13*.

Wolff, S. (2004). The history of autism. *European Child & Adolescent Psychiatry*, *13*(4), 201–208. doi:10.1007/s00787-004-0363-5.

Xu, G., Strathearn, L., Liu, B., et al. (2019). Prevalence and Treatment Patterns of Autism Spectrum Disorder in the United States, 2016. *JAMA Pediatr.* *173*(2), 153–159. doi:10.1001/jamapediatrics.2018.4208.

Yoon, S., Choi, J., Lee, W. and Do, J.T. (2020). Genetic and epigenetic etiology underlying autism spectrum disorder. *Journal of Clinical Medicine*, *9*.

Zwaigenbaum, L., Bryson, S., Brian, J., Smith, I., Roberts, W., Szatmari, P., Roncadin, C., Garon, N. and Vaillancourt, T. (2016). Stability of diagnostic assessment for autism spectrum disorder between 18 and 36 months in a high-risk cohort. *Autism Research*, *9*.

3 Prevailing Diagnostic Scenario and the Importance of Early Detection

Desirée Louise Procópio Alves[1*] and Fabiano Tonaco Borges[2]

Autism spectrum disorder is one of the most relevant medical conditions of our era due to its increasing prevalence and the need for significant medical, educational, and social support. Early diagnosis of autism spectrum disorder is crucial because it allows for appropriate intervention and leads to better long-term outcomes, improved quality of life for patients and their families, and access to educational and community resources. Unfortunately, there are no established screening programs for fetal, prenatal, or neonatal autism, making early detection challenging. Some scales are used as screening tools to facilitate identification, referral to specialists, and diagnosis. However, there are significant challenges in accessing and navigating appropriate services and support, causing high levels of stress and anxiety among families and delaying interventions for the patient. This chapter will discuss the benefits of early detection, the current diagnostic scenario, and the direction research is taking for the incorporation of new approaches.

1. Introduction

Autism Spectrum Disorder (ASD) is a neurodevelopmental disorder characterized by difficulties in social interaction and communication, along with restricted and/or repetitive patterns of behavior and interests. The symptoms and severity of ASD can vary widely from child to child. To meet the definition, these behaviors must appear early in life and cause some level of social impairment. Therefore, current ASD tests and diagnoses are based on the clinical manifestation of the mentioned social, behavioral, and communicative difficulties, and challenges. Detection usually occurs in early childhood, around 18–24 months, partly because abnormal behaviors may not be evident until the disorder is well established and only become fully apparent when social demands exceed the child's capacities. However, early signs may appear before one year of age. ASD has a multifactorial pathogenesis primarily

1 Neuropediatrician, Brazil
2 Universidade Federal de Pernambuco, Brazil.
* Corresponding author: dradesireeneuroped@gmail.com.

DOI: 10.1201/9781003531418-3

due to the interaction of genetic, environmental, biological, psychological, and immunological factors, as well as advanced parental age (Okoye et al., 2023; Al-Beltagi, 2023; Lotan, 2024).

Table 1 Prevalence of Autism Across Selected Countries: Estimates, Gender Ratios, and Intellectual Disability Proportions.

Country	*Prevalence Estimates (per 10,000)*	*Sample Size*	*Gender Ratio (Male: Female)*	*Proportion of Cases with Intellectual Disability (%)*
United States	85 to 284	Variable	4.2:1	33%
Canada	108 to 152	5,100,000	3.9:1	37%
France	47 to 129	1,700,000	4.1:1	38%
China	90 to 135	6,000,000	4.4:1	35%
South Korea	119 to 210	3,500,000	5.1:1	28%
India	50 to 100	4,500,000	4.8:1	40%
Taiwan	110 to 207	1,500,000	5.3:1	32%
Australia	76 to 105	3,200,000	4.5:1	31%
Denmark	68 to 118	2,100,000	4.0:1	35%
Sweden	88 to 140	1,900,000	3.7:1	34%
Spain	95 to 120	2,800,000	4.6:1	36%
Iran	64 to 130	4,000,000	4.9:1	33%
Greece	92 to 108	1,200,000	4.3:1	37%
Israel	101 to 150	1,000,000	4.7:1	38%
Uganda	120 to 205	900,000	5.0:1	29%

Source: Zeidan et al. (2022)

Over the years, there has been an increase in ASD prevalence. This rise is due to various factors, including broader diagnostic criteria and increased risk factors associated with the disorder itself. Table 1 highlights significant variability in autism prevalence estimates across different countries, with rates ranging from as low as 47 per 10,000 in France to as high as 284 per 10,000 in the United States. This variability can be attributed to differences in research methodologies, cultural factors, and the availability of diagnostic resources. Furthermore, the male-to-female ratio consistently shows a higher prevalence of autism in males, with ratios ranging from 3.7:1 to 5.3:1, and the proportion of cases with intellectual disabilities varies significantly, indicating differences in case identification and assessment methods.

Autism spectrum disorder transcends geographical, cultural, and socioeconomic barriers, and these factors influence the availability of resources for treatment as well as how the community deals with the disorder. Early identification provides better prospects, but it is a real challenge due to the heterogeneity of its clinical presentation. It is often difficult to develop a comprehensive diagnostic test that also accounts for specific cultural and social factors of each locality. While the homogeneity of autism may arise from shared failures in the overall socialization process, the heterogeneity may stem from variable timing in the onset of individual disruptions in the reciprocal social interaction between the infant and caregiver (Okoye et al., 2023; Klin et al., 2020).

Given the current demand on the healthcare system for diagnosing and evaluating children with ASD, creating efficient screening systems to better identify those with a higher probability of having ASD becomes valuable (McCarty, P., and Frye, 2020).

2. The Importance of Early Diagnosis

Doctors usually diagnose autism between the ages of two and four because children fully develop social and communicative elements only in the second year of life. Many factors, including the severity of autism, access to healthcare, parental education level, and cultural and community factors, impact the age of diagnosis for autism spectrum disorder. Doctors can diagnose autism at any age, even for the first time during adolescence or adulthood. However, early diagnosis significantly impacts the management, prognosis, and well-being of the child. Therefore, understanding developmental milestones is essential because it allows caregivers to monitor a child's progress in various aspects, including language, communication, cognition, and social and emotional skills. This tool can alert parents and healthcare professionals to developmental delays. Although it does not provide a definitive diagnosis, it indicates that the child needs a formal evaluation (Okoye et al., 2023; Al-Beltagi, 2023).

Early detection is important because a child's brain is still developing. During this time, the brain has a greater capacity for neural organization, allowing interventions to have a more significant impact, better prognosis, and improved quality of life. Targeted actions can slow autism progression, especially in cognitive and language skills, and may even help in the regression of autism due to neuroplasticity.

The first two years of life represent the period of greatest brain transformation. A newborn's brain doubles in size in the first year and will increase by another 35% by the third year. Synaptic density quadruples in the first year alone, with simultaneous pruning and strengthening occurring. Synaptic connections peak between 6–12 months, decreasing drastically after 15 months, which is long before autism symptoms reliably appear and the condition can be diagnosed.

Although there is no accepted timeline for early diagnosis in the literature, age three is considered the limit for early diagnosis. A healthcare system designed to provide treatment only after an ASD diagnosis would miss the best window of opportunity afforded by this initial period of maximum neuroplasticity (Klin et al., 2020).

A definitive diagnosis of autism spectrum disorder requires a full set of necessary signs that likely won't emerge until later in development. By then, an important window of opportunity for early intervention may have been missed. Although autism spectrum disorder has genetic foundations, brain development is not solely guided by an innate genetic timetable for maturation. It also becomes the physical manifestation of the child's experiences, which in turn, moderate epigenetic processes.

Therefore, there is a need for early intervention based on prodromal risks, which are unlikely to be symptoms themselves (such as aberrant behavior) and are more likely to be deviations from normative developmental processes. The longer one waits to intervene and correct the course of an atypical developmental path, such as in ASD, the more entrenched it becomes, and the harder it is to change (Al-Beltagi, 2023; Klin et al., 2020; Girianelli et al., 2023; Kul et al., 2023; Sicherman, 2021). A randomized clinical trial applied preventive intervention for infants showing early behavioral signs of ASD, leading to a significant reduction in the severity of ASD behaviors over the two years between baseline and the study's endpoint at three years of age. This approach reduced the likelihood of an ASD diagnosis in early childhood (Whitehouse et al., 2021).

It is important to note that young children with ASD always differ from their peers in their social attention. When watching complex videos of social situations, typically developing young children will collectively focus on "key points of socialization", or locations on the screen at specific moments in time that carry most of the information they need to process to understand and successfully adapt to the social scene. When measuring these patterns of social visual engagement, moment by moment, young children with ASD differ from their peers hundreds of times in no more than 5–6 minutes of watching videos. These divergences represent missed opportunities for social learning (Klin et al., 2020).

Considering this, several studies have sought to prove this relationship, showing greater social skills and independence in adulthood for those who underwent early intervention. Parents who received an early diagnosis reported lower levels of stress and anxiety, and children who received early interventions showed more significant improvements in cognitive, language, and socio emotional functioning. However, from a public health perspective, the effects of this failure are significant. Due to late detection and diagnosis, at least 50% of children are identified only during the school period, often because of behaviors intensified by years of untreated disorder: severe disruptive behavior and social, communicative, and behavioral symptoms (Girianelli et al., 2023). Considering the economic aspect, the cost of autism can reach up to $3.2 million per person over a lifetime. In this sense, early intervention can improve prognosis and reduce costs, making early detection of autism extremely important (Okoye et al., 2023; Al-Beltagi, 2023).

However, it is not only important to make a diagnosis and offer treatment; involving caregivers is a key element in the treatment of children. While we cannot design a child with "better genes", we can design the type of environment around the child that would probabilistically promote less deviant behavior and more normative behavior. Therefore, there is a need to train and support caregivers so they can use every day experiences to promote socio-communicative development, thereby alleviating the harmful effects of the thousands of missed social learning opportunities experienced by infants and young children with ASD every day (Klin et al., 2020).

The therapeutic intensity of an early intervention is relatively low, and the absence of adverse effects for its broader adoption by the service system are points to be considered. A cost-effectiveness analysis of the entire treatment pathway (incorporating screening and service delivery) and modeling of long-term outcomes in childhood and adulthood are important for determining the feasibility and value of this approach. On the other hand, screening tools designed to identify ASD in young children have high rates of false-positive results, leading to many children being referred for further evaluation who ultimately do not receive an ASD diagnosis. This results in a higher likelihood of receiving medications and behavioral therapies, as well as parental concerns about feeling stigmatized by others and worries about the potential negative impact of labeling on their children's future opportunities and quality of life (Okoye et al., 2023).

3. Current Diagnostic Scenario

ASD was first defined in the third edition of the *Diagnostic and Statistical Manual of Mental Disorders* (*DSM*) in 1980. It is important to note that the diagnostic criteria for autism have changed over time, and what constitutes an autism diagnosis is a subject of ongoing debate among experts. Today, the

DSM-5 is the definitive diagnostic tool and frames autism as a single disorder with a spectrum of severities that must present the following characteristics: impairment in social communication and the presence of repetitive and/or restrictive interests and/or behaviors. However, it describes criteria for diagnosis, including target symptoms, but does not provide a formal assessment for ASD.

For this reason, several instruments have been created to assist in making a diagnosis; however, two are considered the gold standard today: the Autism Diagnostic Observation Schedule (ADOS) and the Autism Diagnostic Interview-Revised (ADI-R). In ADOS, the examiner applies social pressures and observes the subject's response. In the Autism Diagnostic Interview-Revised, a structured interview is conducted with a caregiver based on developmental symptoms and behaviors. These tools require specific training and still have their limitations: caregiver memory and understanding can introduce biases. Diagnosis is typically based on observations and behavioral assessments, and screening tools are not always accurate. These diagnostic tools are very subjective and vary between clinicians. All of these factors together can result in false positives or negatives, leading to overdiagnosis, underdiagnosis, misdiagnosis, or late diagnosis.

Furthermore, autism frequently occurs with many neurological, psychological, and physical comorbidities and overlaps with many other conditions, such as attention deficit hyperactivity disorder, intellectual disability, and language disorders, making differentiation between them difficult (Al-Beltagi, 2023; McCarty and Frye, 2020).

ASD affects approximately 1% of newborns in the European Union, leading to significant social and economic burdens (Fernandez-Lanvin et al., 2024). This condition leads to significant social and economic burdens due to the high dependency levels of affected individuals. The current average age for a definitive ASD diagnosis is around 30 months, even though symptoms may be detectable as early as 18 months. Early intervention is crucial as it can significantly improve the developmental outcomes for children with ASD, reducing their dependency and improving their quality of life. However, the challenge remains in developing objective and automated diagnostic tools that can be used by general pediatricians to identify ASD risk in children under 24 months of age, without relying solely on the expertise of specialized clinicians.

Recent advancements in technology, particularly in eye-tracking devices and machine learning algorithms, offer promising possibilities for the early detection of ASD in young children. The study explores the feasibility of using eye-tracking technology to analyze gaze patterns in toddlers, identifying behavioral markers that distinguish ASD from typically developing children.

By employing a variety of machine learning algorithms, such as Random Forests, Naive Bayes, and Support Vector Machines, the study demonstrates that these methods can achieve high accuracy in diagnosing ASD based on gaze behavior. These technologies have the potential to revolutionize early ASD screening, making it more accessible and less reliant on specialized clinical observations. This approach not only facilitates early intervention but also opens new avenues for research and development in pediatric healthcare, emphasizing the need for further exploration and refinement of automated diagnostic systems.

Despite the benefits of early intervention, late diagnosis is a global reality, with the average age of autism diagnosis in developing countries such as Brazil being higher compared to children diagnosed in other countries. There is also a heterogeneity in the training and distribution of professionals in Brazil and the availability of multidisciplinary teams. In this context, a study concluded that the likelihood of early diagnosis differed among regions, being higher in the Northeast and Southeast than in the North (Girianelli et al., 2023).

Girianelli et al. (2023) also highlighted that, although the early diagnosis of autism and other pervasive developmental disorders has improved in the country, it still accounts for about 30% of diagnoses. They noted that most who received a diagnosis sought specialized care on their own initiative, and referrals from primary care also contributed to early diagnosis. In this study, with a population of up to 12 years, the age of diagnosis ranged from 5.4 years (64.8 months for pervasive developmental disorder) to 6.2 years (74.4 months for atypical autism), while the median age was 5 years (60 months), except for atypical autism, which was higher. Therefore, what can be identified is that the severity of symptoms and access to health and education systems were determining factors for early diagnosis, and the performance of local policies and infrastructure seems to cause differences in diagnostic age between different regions (Girianelli et al., 2023).

It is essential to consider that developing countries with limited financial resources (including Brazil) have limited specialized services. Considering this point, along with the fact that parents generally first approach pediatricians with questions about their child's development, it would be important for pediatricians to be familiar with the early signs of ASD, diagnostic tools, and to provide initial guidance so families can access the necessary resources for managing the child.

Although the American Academy of Pediatrics recommends universal screening for children between 18–24 months, adherence among pediatricians is low. In this context, an excellent screening test is the Modified Checklist for Autism in Toddlers, Revised with Follow-Up (M-CHAT-R/F). This tool has been extensively studied, is free, translated into many languages, and can be completed by parents in 5–10 minutes. It has high sensitivity (91%) and specificity (96%). However, it is important to emphasize that a screening test cannot make a diagnosis, and children should be referred for further evaluation. The American Academy of Neurology (AAN) recommends further investigation for ASD if a child shows a lack of babbling or gestures at 12 months, a single spoken word at 16 months, spontaneous two-word phrases at 24 months, or any loss of language or social skills at any time (McCarty and Frye, 2020; Singhi and Smith-Hicks, 2023; Kopanska et al., 2021).

Other measures, such as promoting education about the topic at all levels of healthcare that deal with children and their families, developing team-based strategies, public-private partnerships, and international collaborations are interesting initiatives. Another aspect to consider is that as the number of working mothers continues to increase, the need for public childcare services also constantly rises. Therefore, daycare caregivers can be seen as some of the most important professionals for many young children. Consequently, it seems important to explore a potential role for daycare caregivers in the early detection of atypical development in young children.

Zhang et al. (2019) suggest that daycare workers are competent in accurately reporting the early signs of autism by applying well-developed behavioral checklists. Among the potential advantages of integrating this help is that these personnel generally have training and knowledge of early child development and have considerable practical experience working with children of comparable ages and diverse developmental profiles. Therefore, it may be important to involve daycare workers as potential screeners for developmental disabilities. To maximize the contribution of daycare professionals in supporting the early identification of atypical development, using a specifically designed checklist of signs and providing related training can be effective and desirable.

Given this, it is possible to observe that education is important in a general sense, as it directly impacts the age of diagnosis. Literature data indicate that sociodemographic aspects directly affect the age of diagnosis through observations such as: children of parents with secondary education or lower are diagnosed later than children of parents with higher education; a larger number of children in the home; and parents who denied the symptoms or symptoms first noticed by others rather than the parents themselves are also related to later diagnoses. Mothers are primarily the ones who observe the first signs (62.4% of cases), compared to fathers (8.9%) and others (teachers, healthcare professionals) in 28.7% of cases (Kul et al., 2023; Sicherman et al., 2021).

In general, the main reason for taking a patient to the doctor is speech delay. Therefore, it is essential to keep an ASD diagnosis in mind in children with speech delays. Another complaint frequently expressed by families with an ASD diagnosis was hyperactivity, poor response to their own name, and lack of gestures. The severity of symptoms is associated with an earlier diagnosis. Most skill regressions, as well as restricted and repetitive behaviors, were also associated with an earlier age of diagnosis, although on a smaller scale. Some studies suggest that the lack of such communication problems in early development may mask social difficulties until later in development, contributing to a delay in the diagnosis of those cases where there was no speech delay. It is important to emphasize that parents observed these symptoms long before the current average age of diagnosis. This suggests the potential value of designing targeted tools that can enable family members to identify the key early symptoms of ASD before they catch the attention of healthcare specialists (Kul et al., 2023; Sicherman et al., 2021).

In this regard, characteristics that occur before the first year of life have been studied to contribute to an earlier diagnosis. Tang et al. (2023) reported the following characteristics occur more frequently in children with ASD:

- Between 9–12 months of age, they respond poorly to their own name and rarely look at the faces of others.
- At 6 months of age, children show a weak response to looking at people.
- From 0 to 6 months of age, they have significantly weaker orientation towards people.
- They spend less time looking at caregivers and more time looking at a toy or video game controller compared to a low-risk group.
- Motor and sensory concerns at 6 months of age were more frequent among parents of children later diagnosed with autism.

In this regard, Kul et al. (2023) and Sicherman et al. (2021) observed that being evaluated by a pediatrician or family doctor in the last six months was also not associated with an early diagnosis. This is an alarming finding that highlights the need for better training in healthcare. In addition to the deficiency related to recognizing signs and providing guidance about ASD, another important contributing factor to this situation may be that doctors cannot allocate sufficient time to patients due to the workload they face. They often focus on the family's complaint and do not find time to conduct a general evaluation (Kul et al., 2023; Singhi and Smith-Hicks, 2023).

Furthermore, it is important to be aware of the risk factors for autism spectrum disorder so that, in their presence, closer monitoring can be provided, and early intervention can be implemented if necessary. Numerous data suggest that ASD may originate from genetic or environmental pathological events occurring in the womb. Some well-established risk factors include advanced parental age, multiple pregnancies, psychosocial stress, certain medical conditions during pregnancy (including infections such as rubella, influenza, cytomegalovirus, measles, chickenpox, toxoplasmosis, urinary tract infection, herpes), celiac disease, premature birth, birth complications, significant pre-pregnancy obesity, vitamin deficiencies (such as vitamin D), and exposure to certain substances (such as cocaine, valproic acid, tobacco, and alcohol) (Kopanska et al., 2021; Ben-Ari et al., 2022).

Traditional statistical approaches are limited in their ability to combine potentially predictive features. However, the effective combination of family history of ASD, prescribed medications, and socioeconomic variables can produce greater predictive power than a single factor alone.

Considering this, machine learning has been studied as a method capable of efficiently combining features derived from large datasets, thus generating clinically relevant predictions. On the other hand, this also raises an ethical issue: the knowledge of a possible ASD diagnosis can be a source of stress for both the parents and the child (Ben-Ari et al., 2022; Rahman et al., 2020). However, aspects such as society's and relatives' perceptions of the disorder can also contribute to delayed diagnosis, directly influenced by factors like region, public policies, education, and others (Singhi and Hicks, 2023).

The conventional diagnostic approaches currently used for ASD, considered the gold standard, include multiple dimensions and generally rely heavily on behavioral assessments and specialist interviews, sometimes requiring additional evaluations such as vision and hearing tests to rule out sensory impairments. These special assessment methods are often subjective or expensive. Therefore, there is an urgent need to develop a safe, convenient, and accurate method for diagnosing ASD.

Although these methods offer cutting-edge diagnoses, their inherent subjectivity, lack of trained professionals, and human bias highlight the need for more objective and effective tools. These tools could also help in tracking what is called pre-autism, an early stage of autism during which signs and symptoms may appear, indicating a potential risk of developing autism later in life. In this regard, various physical, biochemical, hormonal, and imaging biomarkers are being evaluated to assist in the prenatal and early diagnosis of autism. Nonetheless, no single molecular marker defines its diagnosis. Instead, current estimates suggest that hundreds of genetic and genomic disorders (most of which are still unknown) may play a role in its etiology, with some variants being rare and others common (Al-Beltagi, 2023; Klin et al., 2020; Alam et al., 2024).

Considering this, MRI alterations have been extensively studied to review abnormal characteristics in the brain's structural-functional networks, perfusion, neuronal metabolism, and glymphatic system in children with ASD, which may aid in early diagnosis and precise intervention. It was found that the brain volume of children with ASD begins to increase between the ages of 12–24 months, rapidly grows at 2.5 years, and increases by approximately 10% compared to the brains of typically developing children between the ages of 2–4 years. The brain volume then increases slowly during late childhood and adolescence.

Compared to typically developing children, children with autism spectrum disorder have increased volumes in the bilateral superior frontal gyrus (closely associated with social and cognitive deficits), left precuneus, left inferior occipital gyrus, right angular gyrus, bilateral superior temporal gyrus, and left inferior parietal lobule of the brain (while the right inferior temporal gyrus is smaller in volume).

Regarding the hippocampus, it plays an important role in the central functions of the "social brain". Changes in its volume can lead to cognitive and language deficits, with the left hippocampal white matter volume often being larger compared to typically developing children. Previous studies also highlight histopathological changes in the cerebellum (reduction in granule cells, hypertrophy, and atrophy of the cerebellar nuclei can be observed in the post-mortem brains of individuals with ASD).

Changes in cerebellar volume can also predict the emergence of restricted and repetitive behaviors in early childhood and correlate with the severity of motor restrictions. Given all these findings, abnormalities in the prefrontal cortex and cerebellum are suggested as early biomarkers for ASD diagnosis. Additionally, MRI not only reveals morphological differences in brain structures across different age groups but also helps clarify the pathophysiological changes of the disorder by correlating them with the main symptoms of ASD. Wang et al. (2023) believes that MRI contributes to the early diagnosis of ASD.

Notwithstanding, eye-tracking technology has become an increasingly important tool in the early screening and diagnosis of ASD in recent years. In contrast to electroencephalography (EEG) and magnetic resonance imaging (MRI), which are time-consuming and challenging to perform, eye-tracking allows for the investigation of visual exploration patterns and their underlying mechanisms (Meng et al., 2023)

Eye-tracking techniques can be promising in the early and objective diagnosis of ASD, as this disorder is characterized by a decrease in gaze towards stimuli with high social significance and an increase in gaze towards stimuli with low social significance. Meng et al. (2023) found that several gaze behaviors related to real humans or human parts, such as head gaze duration, person gaze count, and time spent fixating on a person, were all negatively associated with ASD. When associating cartoon characters, children were more likely to have ASD if they were less interested in real humans or human parts and more interested in the cartoon characters.

In recent years, pervasive technologies and sensor systems aimed at refining the detection of typical movements and characteristics of individuals with ASD have also garnered interest. This observation would be valuable both for diagnosis and for therapeutic purposes targeting specific behaviors in children with ASD. The prevalence of general motor deficits among people with ASD has ranged from 50% to 80%, with various impairments in basic gross and fine motor skills and motor coordination, resulting in slow, clumsy, or inaccurate motor performance and difficulties in motor learning. Children at risk for ASD exhibit less advanced skills in grasping and handling objects, lower rates of giving objects to others, fewer approaches to caregivers, and lower rates of stepping toward task-appropriate goals compared to typically developing infants in the first year of life.

Lotan (2024), and Bondioli et al. (2021) suggest that infants who were later diagnosed with ASD exhibited greater asymmetry in posture and movement compared to typically developing infants, as well as less rhythmic and weaker body movement patterns at 4 months of age. Since motor development begins during the gestational period and is independent of social or linguistic development, the existence of such motor abnormalities at such a young age is an alarming phenomenon. If such peculiarities exist independently of any connection with social and communicative skills, it suggests that motor deficits are present in infants with ASD from birth. This abnormality raises the possibility that motor issues are a key element in ASD.

Given this, motor difficulties are a significant issue for children diagnosed with ASD, and they do not disappear with age. By around 9–12 years of age, children diagnosed with ASD perform motor tasks at the level of children half their age. This device could also aid in detecting repetitive behaviors. Motor assessments are a promising tool, as the motor signs exhibited by infants later diagnosed with ASD can be observed well before subsequent behavioral, communicative, or social symptoms can be detected.

The results of interventional studies (Lotan, 2024; Bondioli et al., 2021) also show that motor interventions improve the core symptoms of ASD, in some cases with modest long-term effects. Since motor and sensory elements influence each other, early diagnosis (at 2–4 months of age), primarily based on motor signs, followed by early sensory-physical interventions (therapy), can be effectively implemented at the early age of several months. This approach has the potential to reduce future ASD symptoms and increase the ability of individuals with ASD to integrate into society. However, for clinical and research purposes, more accessible and reliable computational measures of motor performance are needed.

In addition to motor sensors, the measurement of auditory sensory responses has also been a field of interest. The Brainstem Auditory Evoked Response (BAER) test, an auditory evoked potential that measures the electrical signals from the brainstem in response to a sound, has been used. The response is recorded by surface electrodes and results in a succession of different waves (I–V). In autistic children aged two to six years, wave I shows greater amplitude than wave V, which is the opposite of what is observed in neurotypical children. Differences in electrical responses have also been observed in newborns: those who were later diagnosed with ASD exhibited a delayed response to sounds compared to other newborns.

Other approaches have been tested, particularly the exploration of facial reactions, which appear to take longer in children with ASD, along with an atypical exploratory process, or the perception of language and voice. Despite their potential role in understanding developmental changes in children with ASD and as biomarkers in these children, it is unlikely that such approaches would become established as diagnostic tools that can be used with newborns in the general population (Ben-Ari et al., 2022).

Regarding biomarkers, they may be promising, as many studies have shown that oxidative stress plays a crucial role in the process of ASD because cases exhibit higher levels of oxidative stress and reduced antioxidant capacity. The active use of biomarkers could be used to monitor the physiological state of patients with ASD and be useful for the diagnosis, intervention, and treatment of the disorder. Although many potential oxidative stress markers have been identified in ASD, attempts to monitor the oxidative stress state in children with ASD still struggle to meet clinical application standards, particularly due to significant individual differences, indicating that ASD is heterogeneous. Therefore, additional studies are necessary for their practical implementation (Liu et al., 2022).

Another existing field of study is related to genetics, as research has shown that ASD is highly hereditary. However, at present, genetic screening cannot reliably predict ASD. For example, despite progress in identifying rare genetic variants associated with ASD, single-gene disorders account for only 3–7% of all ASD cases, so genetic screening has limited utility in families with idiopathic ASD. Taken together, risk assessment models based solely on genetic information do not function reliably in the context of ASD's complex etiology (Rahman, 2020).

Although associated comorbidities can sometimes make differentiation difficult, different authors emphasize the importance of performing a phenotypic characterization based not only on the core symptoms specific to ASD but also on its psychiatric and medical comorbidities and other factors that may influence the functionality of this complex autism spectrum. This approach can aid in early identification. These associations suggest structural and functional neuroimaging differences in autism, as previously mentioned, with one of the most well-known associations being the high risk of epilepsy due to CNS (central nervous system) dysfunction.

In the literature, the reported prevalence of epilepsy in patients with ASD ranges from 2.4% to 46%. According to Roberto Tuchman, the concept of an epileptiform disorder with cognitive symptoms includes a subgroup of individuals with ASD who present epileptiform abnormalities in EEG results in the absence of clinical seizures. Additionally, several studies have demonstrated the impact of epileptiform abnormalities on the developing brain, even when seizures are absent. Other authors have also shown that epileptiform abnormalities in children with ASD are associated with a higher level of motor stereotypes, more aggressive behavior symptoms, language deficits, lower adaptive functioning, cognitive function, and other sociodemographic and clinical variables, such as age and diagnostic classification.

The presence of intellectual disability has been reported as an independent risk factor for the development of epilepsy in the context of ASD. Early detection of abnormalities in EEG signals may serve as an early biomarker for developmental or coexisting cognitive disorders. However, further research is needed to investigate whether these EEG abnormalities are an epiphenomenon or play a more direct role in some of the characteristics observed in ASD (Romero-González et al., 2022).

4. Conclusion

Multiple factors make the early detection of autism a significant challenge. Despite increased awareness of the condition, there is still a frequent lack of knowledge about its signs and symptoms among parents, family members, caregivers, and even healthcare professionals, which is one of the main obstacles to early detection. Another critical challenge is the variability in symptoms. Autism is a complex and common neurodevelopmental disorder that affects children differently, with a wide range of symptoms and levels of severity. Symptoms also vary depending on the child's age, sex, and cultural background.

Another essential point is to challenge the perception that autism spectrum disorder inevitably brings burdens, with only improvements offering some relief from symptoms and an increase in independent living skills. Unless reconciled by the emerging science of gene-brain-behavior interdependencies in the neuroscience of early brain development, there is a concern that the world of opportunities enabled by early detection and early treatment will remain underdeveloped.

References

Al-Beltagi, M. (2023). Pre-autism: What a paediatrician should know about early diagnosis of autism. *World Journal of Clinical Pediatrics*, *12*(5): 273–294.

Alam, M.S., Elsheikh, E.A.A., Suliman, F.M., Rashid, M.M. and Faizabadi, A.R. (2024). Innovative strategies for early autism diagnosis: Active learning and domain adaptation optimization. *Diagnostics*, *14*(6).

Ben-Ari, Y., Caly, H., Rabiei, H. and Lemonnier, É. (2022). Early prognostic of ASD: A challenge. *Médecine/Sciences*, *38*, 431–437. Editions EDK.

Bondioli, M., Chessa, S., Narzisi, A., Pelagatti, S. and Zoncheddu, M. (2021). Towards motor-based early detection of autism red flags: Enabling technology and exploratory study protocol. *Sensors*, *21*(6), 1–15.

Fernandez-Lanvin, D., Gonzalez-Rodriguez, M., De-Andres, J. and Camero, R. (2024). Towards an automatic early screening system for autism spectrum disorder in toddlers based on eye-tracking. *Multimedia Tools and Applications*, *83*(3), 55319–55350. https://doi.org/10.1007/s11042-023-17694-8.

Girianelli, V.R., Tomazelli, J., da Silva, C.M.F.P. and Fernandes, C.S. (2023). Early diagnosis of autism and other developmental disorders, Brazil, 2013–2019. *Revista de Saúde Pública*, *57*. https://doi.org/10.11606/s1518-8787.2023057004351.

Klin, A., Micheletti, M., Klaiman, C., Shultz, S., Constantino, J.N. and Jones, W. (2020). Affording autism an early brain development re-definition. *Development and Psychopathology*, *32*(4), 1175–1189. https://doi.org/10.1017/S0954579420000782.

Kopanska, M., Ochojska, D., Banas-Zabczyk, A., Sochocka, M., Ochnik, M., Torices, S., et al. (2021). Brain as the house of autistic soul: Current trends in analyzing the risk factors and building up the diagnosis in mild forms of autism spectrum disorder. *Journal of Physiology and Pharmacology*, *72*(1), 1–10. https://doi.org/10.26402/jpp.2021.1.01.

Kul, M., Dağ, P., Akdağ, B. and Kara, M.Z. (2023). Sociodemographic and social barriers to early detection of autism. *Turkish Journal of Pediatrics*, *65*(5), 778–788. https://doi.org/10.24953/turkjped.2023.05.012.

Liu, X., Lin, J., Zhang, H., Khan, N.U., Zhang, J., Tang, X., et al. (2022). Oxidative stress in autism spectrum disorder: Current progress of mechanisms and biomarkers. *Frontiers in Psychiatry*, *13*. https://doi.org/10.3389/fpsyt.2022.938736.

Lotan, M. (2024). Barking up the wrong tree: Motor–sensory elements as prodrome in autism. *Biomedicines*, *12*(6), 1235.

McCarty, P. and Frye, R.E. (2020). Early detection and diagnosis of autism spectrum disorder: Why is it so difficult? *Seminars in Pediatric Neurology*, *35*, 100831. https://doi.org/10.1016/j.spen.2020.100831.

Meng, F., Li, F., Wu, S., Yang, T., Xiao, Z., Zhang, Y., et al. (2023). Machine learning-based early diagnosis of autism according to eye movements of real and artificial faces scanning. *Frontiers in Neuroscience*, *17*. https://doi.org/10.3389/fnins.2023.00256.

Okoye, C., Obialo-Ibeawuchi, C.M., Obajeun, O.A., Sarwar, S., Tawfik, C., Waleed, M.S., et al. (2023). Early diagnosis of autism spectrum disorder: A review and analysis of the risks and benefits. *Cureus*.

Rahman, R., Kodesh, A., Levine, S.Z., Sandin, S., Reichenberg, A. and Schlessinger, A. (2020). Identification of newborns at risk for autism using electronic medical records and machine learning. *European Psychiatry*, *63*(1). https://doi.org/10.1192/j.eurpsy.2020.36.

Romero-González, M., Navas-Sánchez, P., Marín-Gámez, E., Barbancho-Fernández, M.A., Fernández-Sánchez, V.E., Lara-Muñoz, J.P., et al. (2022). EEG abnormalities and clinical phenotypes in pre-school children with autism spectrum disorder. *Epilepsy and Behavior*, *129*. https://doi.org/10.1016/j.yebeh.2022.108549.

Sicherman, N., Charite, J., Eyal, G., Janecka, M., Loewenstein, G., Law, K., et al. (2021). Clinical signs associated with earlier diagnosis of children with autism spectrum disorder. *BMC Pediatrics*, *21*(1). https://doi.org/10.1186/s12887-021-02962-1.

Singhi, P. and Smith-Hicks, C. (2023). Early diagnosis and management of autism spectrum disorder (ASD) in low-resource countries: Challenges and strategies. *Indian Journal of Pediatrics*, *90*(5), 362–363. https://doi.org/10.1007/s12098-022-04249-1.

Tang, H., Liang, J., Chai, K., Gu, H., Ye, W., Cao, P., et al. (2023). Artificial intelligence and bioinformatics analyze markers of children's transcriptional genome to predict autism spectrum disorder. *Frontiers in Neurology*, *14*. https://doi.org/10.3389/fneur.2023.00268.

Wang, M., Xu, D., Zhang, L. and Jiang, H. (2023). Application of multimodal MRI in the early diagnosis of autism spectrum disorders: A review. *Diagnostics*, *13*. https://doi.org/10.3390/diagnostics13020364.

Whitehouse, A.J.O., Varcin, K.J., Pillar, S., Billingham, W., Alvares, G.A., Barbaro, J., et al. (2021). Effect of preemptive intervention on developmental outcomes among infants showing early signs of autism: A randomized clinical trial of outcomes to diagnosis. *JAMA Pediatrics*, *175*(11), 1092–1101. https://doi.org/10.1001/jamapediatrics.2021.3349.

Zeidan, J., Fombonne, E., Scorah, J., Ibrahim, A., Durkin, M.S., Saxena, S., Yusuf, A., Shih, A. and Elsabbagh, M. (2022). Global prevalence of autism: A systematic review update. *Autism Research*, *15*(6), 778–790. https://doi.org/10.1002/aur.2696.

Zhang, D., Krieber-Tomantschger, I., Poustka, L., Roeyers, H., Sigafoos, J., Bölte, S., et al. (2019). Identifying atypical development: A role of day-care workers? *Journal of Autism and Developmental Disorders*, *49*(9), 3685–3694.

4 Autism and the DIR/Floortime Model
A Counterpart to Approaches That do not Address Human Singularity

Carol Mota[1*] and Marina Assis Pinheiro[2]

This chapter explores the evolution of therapeutic and educational approaches for autistic individuals. It emphasizes the importance of moving beyond behavior-focused methods to holistic practices that prioritize uniqueness, subjectivity, and human connections. Autism is understood as a neurodevelopmental condition with diverse impacts on sensory, motor, emotional, and communicative aspects. It requires a nuanced perspective that values the unique developmental paths of each individual. By critiquing reductionist methods, including early behaviorist interventions, the study highlights the limitations of prioritizing behavior modification over fostering meaningful engagement and emotional co-regulation. Our approach builds on the Developmental, Individual-difference, Relationship-based (DIR) model and its application through DIR/Floortime. It advocates for practices rooted in affectivity, sensory-motor understanding, and communication. It emphasizes the role of relationships and natural contexts in promoting learning and development while addressing ethical concerns tied to traditional methodologies. Through a discussion of theoretical foundations, including insights from Vygotsky and contemporary critiques, the study underscores the importance of respecting autistic individuals' temporalities and intentionalities. It calls for inclusive, dialogical environments that embrace diversity and support autonomy. These environments should advance therapeutic and educational practices that humanize and empower autistic individuals and their families. This approach fosters not just skill development but holistic well-being and meaningful participation in society.

1. Introduction

This chapter aims to explain the DIR/Floortime model and offer a critical reflection on approaches that disregard the uniqueness of autistic individuals. It

[1] PhD in Cognitive Psychology, Master's in Education, Cultures, and Identities; DIR/Floortime Therapist.

[2] PhD in Psychology, Department of Psychology, Professor at the Federal University of Pernambuco.

* Corresponding author: mota@hotmail.com.br

DOI: 10.1201/9781003531418-4

calls for inclusive, dialogical environments that embrace diversity and support autonomy. These environments should advance therapeutic and educational practices that humanize and empower autistic individuals and their families.

Since the 1940s, research on autism has provided significant insights across various fields. In 1943, child psychiatrist Leo Kanner[1] introduced the term "early infantile autism", distinguishing it as a unique neurodevelopmental condition separate from psychosis or early schizophrenia, which were common misdiagnoses at the time. Since then, research on autism has significantly advanced, offering valuable insights across multiple fields. The American Psychiatric Association classified autism as a neurodevelopmental disorder and referred to it as Autism Spectrum Disorder (ASD) in the fifth edition of the *Diagnostic and Statistical Manual of Mental Disorders* (*DSM-5*), published in 2013.

Autism is defined as a neurodevelopmental disorder present from early childhood, characterized by deficits in two key areas: social communication and behavior. In 2022, nine years after publishing the *DSM-5*, professionals completed the *DSM-5-TR* revision. This updated version keeps the same core criteria that the *DSM-5* (2013) outlines. The latest edition lists the primary diagnostic criteria (F.84) as follows: (I) deficits persist in social communication and interaction across various contexts; (II) behavior, interests, or activities follow restricted and repetitive patterns; (III) symptoms appear during early developmental stages; (IV) symptoms impair functioning in social, occupational, or other critical areas; (V) No other diagnosis explains this condition better.

This classification clarifies and standardizes the diagnosis and treatment of autism spectrum disorder by professionals. *DSM-5-TR* (2022) categorizes levels of support based on individual needs: Level 3 (requiring very substantial support), Level 2 (requiring substantial support), and Level 1 (requiring support) (pp. 212– 215).

To provide readers with diagnostic markers of the condition, the focus outlined above centers on the medical-diagnostic field. However, we believe it is essential to highlight these issues to contribute to the construction of a historical-social perspective on autism. The medical model and the social model represent two distinct approaches to understanding and addressing disability. The medical model views disability as a limitation that must be overcome, focusing primarily on the individual's deficit in meeting societal norms or

1 Leo Kanner (1894–1981) was a pioneering child psychiatrist known for his seminal work in identifying and describing "early infantile autism" in 1943. His paper, *Autistic Disturbances of Affective Contact*, differentiated autism as a distinct neurodevelopmental condition, laying the foundation for modern understanding and research on Autism Spectrum Disorder (ASD).

expectations due to their condition. In contrast, the social model emphasizes the social and environmental barriers that hinder the full participation of people with disabilities in society.

While acknowledging the DSM's contributions to the historical study of ASD, we aim to move away from the medical perspective and focus on the uniqueness of the individual.

In this chapter, we understand autism as a neurodevelopmental condition. This means that the brain, embodiment, and subjectivity of a person on the autism spectrum differ from those of a neurotypical person within a sociocultural context.

Such differences significantly impact a person's development in various areas. From this perspective, the term 'neurodivergent' is used to refer to individuals whose neurological functioning is marked by an intense singularity. We avoid using certain classifications, such as high-functioning and low-functioning, mild, moderate, and severe autism, or support levels 1, 2, and 3. These labels are considered reductionist and limiting because they focus solely on functioning, overlooking the individual's subjectivity and potential as a human being.

Throughout the decades following the 1940s, various intervention models for autistic individuals emerged, aiming to provide a foundation for teaching and learning practices in therapeutic and educational contexts. Two fundamental perspectives stand out: behavioral and developmental. These theoretical frameworks guide therapeutic and educational practices, emphasizing the need for models that serve as markers, given that practices in psychology and education do not occur without a theoretical basis. These models offer possibilities and pathways for services provided to autistic individuals.

Historically, the approach rooted in the study of observable actions, known as Behaviorism, rose to significant prominence in work with autistic children. With its primary focus on behavioral changes, this approach became the most widely disseminated. However, recognizing the limitations of this perspective in addressing developmental issues, Stanley Greenspan (1941–2010) introduced the DIR/Floortime model in the 1980s. This approach offered a new way of understanding development, sensitive to the complexities inherent to autism. The developmental perspective focuses on how individuals organize their experiences at different developmental stages, considering their uniqueness, affective experiences, and relational context.

Development and learning are topics that must connect with comprehensive therapeutic and educational models. These models should foster dialogue and reflection through respectful practices that consider everyone's uniqueness in the learning process. Acting from a respectful perspective with autistic individuals requires understanding their development and underlying processes to enable learning to occur in an enjoyable and healthy way. A respectful perspective values the emancipation of thought, the individual's unique temporality, and autonomy. It also preserves uniqueness as a hallmark of human potential and a fundamental ethical premise regarding the unique condition of every human being.

The notion of uniqueness allows us to understand why each person has a unique perspective on the world. Uniqueness is inherent but also constructed in relationships with others, always recognizing other ways of being, existing, and other points of view. Each event exists in correlation with the individual's singularity, even though some aspects are part of their structure and responsiveness. When we address uniqueness, we recognize that individuals may share the same condition but exhibit unique characteristics. It is essential to understand how each one responds to the world.

When we focus on uniqueness, we aim not to obscure a person's subjectivity with the diagnosis they carry. Many practices and studies in the therapeutic and educational fields involving individuals on the autism spectrum tend to focus solely on traits associated with the spectrum, rather than valuing uniqueness.

By focusing on the defining characteristics of a disorder and overlooking individual subjectivity, they adopt a de-subjectivizing approach—one that underscores what a hegemonic and homogeneous society deems 'different'. This perspective hinders the learning and development of autistic individuals in relation to others.

The approach we advocate stems from the developmental perspective and emphasizes uniqueness. We highlight the importance of this perspective in working with autistic individuals, where the DIR/Floortime model offers an alternative to approaches that neglect individuality. It fosters practices that recognize and respect the unique traits of each person. We begin with a reflection on the philosophical premises, addressing the epistemological and ontological foundations that enable understanding contemporary approaches. Next, we discuss the origins of the DIR/Floortime model and its contributions to the development and learning of autistic individuals. By sharing observations and reflections on traditional, hegemonic practices, we seek to bring these concepts to life and foster the development of more humane, sensitive approaches that honor each autistic individual's uniqueness.

2. Philosophical Foundations of Psychological Theories

As a starting point for building new knowledge, epistemology and ontology standpoints are crucial. They help us understand the philosophical and psychological contributions underlying this chapter.

Epistemology is the theory or study of knowledge—it can be described as a reflective study of knowing, including its organization, formation, functioning, and development, as well as its possibilities and limitations. Ontology, on the other hand, refers to the philosophical perspectives concerning the nature of being and existence (Bunge, 1980).

Without an ontological foundation, psychology would be incapable of establishing the premises for theoretical and phenomenological constructs. Thus, engaging in dialogue with the field of philosophy is vital to broaden our understanding of humanness, the world, and the psychological universe in a more comprehensive and profound way.

Until the second half of the 19th century, the study of human nature was the domain of philosophy—the field from which psychology emerged. Many philosophers explored questions related to psychology and human development. Numerous themes in contemporary psychology were originally subjects of philosophical debate. This historical interplay contributed to the emergence of a wide variety of perspectives within psychology and education.

The organismic model, pioneered by Rousseau, views individuals as active, growing organisms that initiate events rather than merely react to them. As a result, the force driving change is internal. Since human behavior is perceived as a cohesive, organic whole, it cannot be predicted by breaking it down into simple responses to environmental stimuli.

For organismic theorists, development has an underlying and ordered structure. They describe postnatal development as a progressive sequence of stages leading toward full maturation. These theorists support stage theories, where development occurs through distinct stages, each fundamentally different from the previous one. Early stages provide the foundation for later ones, and skipping stages is not considered possible. Many scholars regard these processes as universal, explaining human development across all contexts, though specific timelines may vary slightly.

Over the centuries, much of philosophers' thinking has transformed. Theoretical perspectives have evolved, giving rise to new practices rooted in these initial views on development and the child's role in the learning process. All theories of development and learning carry implicit assumptions. These influence the methods used, the ways of teaching, and the interpretation of data.

Behaviorism (behavior = behavior) states that individuals are reactive, and that the environment regulates behavior. It does not operate through stages. It treats experience casually and views the individual as reactive in the learning process. The cognitive sociocultural perspective holds that social interaction drives cognitive development. It proceeds through stages, places emphasis on experience, and regards the individual as active in learning (Papalia, 2022).

Considering this, two main conceptions currently stand out in services provided for autistic individuals: behavioral and developmental. Norwegian psychologist Ivar Lovaas (1927–2010) began working with autistic children in the 1960s, focusing on conditioning neurotypical behaviors. Behaviorism, which views learning as a form of conditioning, underpins his approach, now commonly known as Applied Behavior Analysis (ABA).

ABA observes, analyzes, and explains the relationship between the environment, human behavior, and learning. For autistic individuals, ABA-based interventions focus on teaching new skills, addressing challenging behaviors, and enhancing communication.

A few years later, in the 1980s, the developmental perspective introduced the DIR/Floortime model, offering a new outlook on development and the learning process.

3. The Birth of the DIR/Floortime Model and Its Contributions to the Development and Learning of Autistic Individuals

Following behavioral interventions that focused solely on the behavior of autistic children, Stanley Greenspan—a clinical professor, physician, and psychiatrist—emphasized the need for a natural, uncontrolled environment. He introduced developmental intervention as a new alternative. In the 1980s, Greenspan and Serena Wieder—a psychologist with a Ph.D. in psychology—combined insights from various studies on child development, recognizing the importance of relationships and emotional connections in learning.

The DIR/Floortime model emerged rooted in the science of human development and grounded in a socio constructivist approach. This contrasts with behavioral methods based on the behaviorist perspective. DIR serves as a comprehensive framework for understanding human development, while DIR/Floortime, or simply Floortime, applies the DIR framework in practice, providing tools to promote developmental progress.

In the DIR model, 'D' addresses functional and emotional developmental capacities. 'I' refers to individual differences. Each person perceives the world in a unique way and processes sensory information—such as sounds, touch, smells, and movement—differently. These variations shape their relationships, actions, and thoughts. Meanwhile, 'R' underscores the importance of human relationships.

The central goal of the DIR model is to build a healthy foundation for social, emotional, and cognitive capacities rather than focusing solely on isolated skills and behaviors. DIR/Floortime has become widely recognized as an approach to supporting autistic children. It is a dialogical model—occurring through a continuous exchange of meanings between the individual and others—that respects and holistically understands the person while addressing their specific needs. The model works collaboratively with families, emphasizing the child's emotional and interactional needs. It uses the child's interests to build and expand their developmental progress through play.

Greenspan and Wieder (2006) emphasize that the behavioral approach fails to account for the unique way each individual responds to the world. It lacks a specific focus on the individual's unique traits, including how they process sensory stimuli, plan and sequence actions, and express themselves. They maintain that knowledge arises from real-world experiences rather than memorizing facts, emphasizing that emotion drives behavior. Regarding autistic children, they highlight how the myth "they cannot learn" has inspired some interventions built around repetitive activities to teach specific skills.

The DIR model rejects generalizations and designs a unique intervention for each individual based on their specific characteristics. Lampreia (2007) notes that the DIR model

> [...] aims to enable the child to develop a sense of self as an intentional, interactive individual and to cultivate linguistic and social capacities. It considers developmental skills such as attention and focus, engagement and social relationships, non-verbal gestures, affect, problem-solving, symbolic communication, abstract thinking, and logical reasoning. These skills are referred to as functional emotional processes because they are rooted in early emotional interactions (Lampreia, 2007).

Intentionality is a key aspect of the DIR model, guiding interactive exchanges. Instead of ignoring them, we acknowledge the individual's actions and use them to guide interactive exchanges, with emotional engagement forming the foundation of this process. For this reason, DIR is action-oriented rather than behavior-oriented. By observing the child's interests and intentions, the adult follows the child's lead during interactions, building bridges that foster interactive exchanges. This approach aims to sustain engagement and expand cognitive, socio-communicative, sensory-motor, problem-solving, and symbolic skills, among others.

Greenspan and Wieder (2006) proposed that the adult's role is to participate in activities initiated by the child, using play as a guide to expand interactions. This approach contrasts significantly with the adult-centric perspective in behavioral interventions. In those interventions, the adult defines appropriate behaviors and dictates the learning context rather than following the child's leadership, interests, and motivations. Following the child's natural interests means discovering the essence of their motivation. What does the child enjoy doing? Instead of relying on preconceived notions or thinking about 'rewards', it is essential to follow their interests.

Floortime, the practice of following the child's interests and leadership, allows the child to guide play while the adult participates in the interaction by validating and supporting their intentionality. Similarly, the DIR model and Floortime allow us to follow the interests and directions of adolescents and adults.

> For children, the process of engaged, spontaneous, and developmentally appropriate interaction is called "Floortime". For adults, a similar approach may be referred to as "Intentional Interaction" or "Coregulation". Affect, when experienced within the context of regulated and emotionally attuned relationships with others, forms the foundation for helping children and adults with developmental and processing challenges experience "coregulation". This process involves learning to manage internal states through shared subjectivity and the contingent responses of a caring other. Coregulation serves as the foundation for therapeutic effectiveness in the DIR model and Floortime interventions (Christian, 2011, p. 25).

The use of relationship-based approaches with adolescents and adults acknowledges the ongoing strength of primary relationships throughout human life, which affect and influence individual growth. Since 2011, several randomized controlled studies have compared DIR/Floortime with traditional behavioral approaches. These studies have highlighted significant advancements for autistic children (Solomon et al., 2014; Casenhiser, Shanker, and Steiben, 2011; Lal and Chhabria, 2013; Pajareya and Kopmaneejumruslers, 2011; Pajareya et al., 2019). Most of these studies also examined parental stress, finding that the DIR/Floortime approach significantly reduced this stress factor.

In an article published in the *Journal of the American Medical Association* (2020) titled "Intervention Recommendations for Autistic Children in Light of a Changing Evidence Base", Sandbank et al. recommended that pediatricians explore and suggest a broader range of options for families, considering that,

> There has been a recent and sharp increase in both the quantity and quality of research examining interventions for young children with autism. Between 2011 and 2018, the reported number of randomized controlled trials (RCTs) on interventions for young children with autism rose from 2 to 48. To summarize this transformative evidence base, we systematically reviewed and meta-analyzed 150 reports from 130 studies, including 87 RCTs,

> which collectively reported effect sizes for 1,615 outcomes, representing 6,240 young children with autism. Several findings emerged from this research, but two are of direct relevance to pediatricians guiding families toward services and supports after a diagnosis. First, three intervention approaches that are not currently widely recommended received more substantial empirical support from RCTs compared to behavioral interventions. These are naturalistic developmental behavioral interventions (NDBIs) and developmental interventions. While distinct from one another, these interventions share commonalities: they are delivered within children's natural contexts (e.g., everyday interactions with caregivers), and their learning targets are guided by early developmental sequences. These attributes may make them preferable for families, as they are less likely to disrupt and separate children from family routines compared to more structured clinician-led interventions (Sandbank et al., 2020).

In 2023, the American Medical Association (AMA) debated and issued a new policy, Resolution 706, altering its stance on support for ABA. Previously, the AMA explicitly supported ABA, but the updated text stated that: "The AMA supports coverage and reimbursement for evidence-based treatment of autism spectrum disorder, including, but not limited to, Applied Behavior Analysis Therapy" (American Medical Association, 2023, pp. 1179–1182).

With this change, the new policy removed direct support for ABA and created room to support evidence-based services, including DIR. Additionally, the AMA shifted away from the term 'treatment' and adopted the term 'services', which is far more appropriate given that autistic individuals may require support from various services. The term 'treatment' implies "fixing the autistic person", a concept that is inadequate and, under societal progress, needs to be revised as it disregards their uniqueness.

In Brazil, the developmental approach has yet to be widely disseminated. Nonetheless, some studies have explored the DIR/Floortime model with autistic children (Araujo, 2023; Lampreia, 2007; Leal, 2018; Solomon, 2013).

Nowadays, child-rearing methods, educational strategies, and social, physical, and mental health services often overlook individual differences, focusing instead on behavior. What drives this focus?

For various reasons that are not yet fully understood—possibly related to chaotic environments or early exposure to substances and habits harmful to the nervous system—children seem to be exhibiting their individual differences with striking clarity. Additionally, over the years, it has become evident that behavioral approaches are insufficient, leaving significant gaps in addressing the complexity of human beings and their development.

In the education of autistic individuals, focusing on individual differences, rather than merely on behaviors, shifts attention to central processes that are fundamental to learning. These include auditory processing and language, visuospatial thinking, motor planning and sequencing (executive function), and sensory modulation. These aspects are crucial because individuals need to develop various levels of abstract thinking, which are essential not only in educational contexts but also in social and emotional interactions. Traditional approaches often overlook these individual differences or the fundamental processing capacities that underpin learning and education, instead emphasizing memorization.

DIR offers a pathway to promote healthy development respectfully through connections, understanding, intersubjective attunement, communication, and engagement.

4. Experienced Materiality: Observations and Reflections on Behavioral Practices

We learn in intersubjective relationships with others and the world. Our affective interactions anchor this process. We do not merely replicate behaviors in an environment. Desires and feelings direct our attention. When we respect a child's interests and pleasures, we strengthen their intention. We guide their actions naturally and affirm their sense of purpose. Desires and emotions must connect with actions and thoughts to build a strong foundation for creative and logical thought.

For example, when a young child is learning to greet someone, relational experiences allow them to associate the act of greeting with feelings of friendship and warmth. This connection leads them to respond to friendly faces with a verbal 'Hi!' If the child perceives a different emotional reaction, such as caution or distrust, they are more likely to look away or hide behind someone who provides a sense of safety. It is affectivity that guides the child's decision to greet or not greet an unfamiliar person.

Encourage discernment about who deserves interaction. Children must learn not to greet strangers in dangerous situations, such as a secluded alley. If a child wants to say "Hi" to someone, that often indicates the person conveys a positive feeling. Children who feel comfortable doing so grow more confident when they meet new people who foster a similar feeling (Greenspan, 2000; Brazelton and Greenspan, 2002).

A child who learned to say: "Good afternoon!" and "Good morning!" every time they entered their building through stimulus-response conditioning, they once said: "Good afternoon!" on a day when no one was at the front desk. This demonstrates a conditioned, non-discriminatory, memorized, and nonreflective action. If children do not connect words with feelings but merely memorize them, abstract words like 'happy' and 'sad' may lack deep meaning. This happens because the continuous process of assigning meaning to words occurs through affective experiences. Each new emotional experience related to a word or concept broadens its meaning.

Words, actions, and shared affects shape and expand our language. Each child relies on emotions to move from familiar to new situations and to decide when and what to say. When we focus on greetings through conditioning alone, without affectivity, we do not help the child generalize or integrate learning. A child who feels angry might, at another moment, display obedience and passivity.

> At yet another time, they might behave competitively or act in a disorganized manner. Thus, an internal emotion such as humiliation and anger can manifest in four or five different ways, depending on contextual situations or other related internal states the child is experiencing. In summary, the principle of multiple determination suggests that there are multiple relationships between what therapists observe and how children organize their experiential world (Greenspan, 1993, p. 12).

We must focus on children's well-being to ensure their learning experiences bring joy, satisfaction, and pleasure. We create a healthy educational environment by establishing guiding boundaries and offering affectionate care. Trust and nurturing relationships help children feel secure and comfortable in their surroundings. These elements foster emotional connections, reduce anxiety, improve communication, promote autonomy, and support learning. When we set boundaries and organize the environment, children learn to regulate their behavior and emotions.

The ability for self-observation arises from the capacity to observe oneself and others within a relationship. Sharing the joy of playing together and solving problems is far more enjoyable than answering questions like "What is this?", "What color is this?", or "What animal is this?". We teach children to think by playing with them, not through questions and answers or memorization cards. Play is where action and development occur during the early years of life. Children require sensitive and nurturing care to build trusting relationships. Later, as they grow, there will be plenty of time to focus on acquiring facts.

We must begin with the child's activity to understand how they think. Through play, the child acts within a cognitive space rather than relying on external, visual cues. They depend on internal motivations and tendencies instead of external incentives from objects.

Before gaining control over their own behavior, the child begins to influence their environment through speech. This not only builds a new organization of their behavior but also creates new relationships with their surroundings (Vygotsky, 2007).

Important concepts in cognitive psychology include perception, memory, attention, language, problem-solving, and executive function. As higher processes develop, the entire structure of behavior shifts. Higher forms of behavior arise from necessity. If there is no need to think, the individual will not think. Culture provides external elements for the child to internalize, and this internalization reshapes all the child's behavior. It opens a new path for development. When delving into Vygotskian thought on defectology:

> We can observe the contrast in Vygotsky's perspective on children with disabilities and their potential to learn. This contrasts with the reductionist conception of their capabilities found in approaches that focus heavily on behavior modification. Vygotsky invites us to overcome, break away from, and transcend mechanized teaching practices and the conditioned formation of habits and merely functional skills, advocating for a broader understanding (Orrú, 2016, p. 158).

We know that culture provides the tools to organize and understand our world in a communicable way. However, individuals are not mere reflections of culture. They interact with it and are also shaped by their own histories. It is always within a socio-historical-cultural context that people relate to and internalize new learning. The expansion of cognitive skills occurs through interactions between self, others, and the world. It is through this process that subjectivity is constructed. The participation of all individuals in culture—engaging and sharing in various activities—is crucial for individual development. Only through this dialogical construction can collectivity be achieved.

Human behavior differs from animal behavior in the same way that human adaptability and development differ from those of animals. The psychological growth of individuals stems from the larger historical development of our species. We must understand it in that context. Embracing this idea calls for a holistic view of psychological phenomena.

Through tools and signs, human behavior transforms nature. This reaction is complex. We cannot study it in an automated way, as if it were a mere object. Instead, we must see it as a living process in constant motion.

Development is a complex, dialectical process. Any learning situation faced by an autistic individual always has a prior history and can never be reduced simply to the formation of skills. When a child explores, interacts, plays, and acts in the world, we witness an opportunity to identify their motivation and expand their engagement with others and their environment. Motivation fundamentally involves observing what the child enjoys and building upon that natural interest to help them learn what they need.

Discover what the child naturally enjoys and use that interest to guide a more personalized, comprehensive approach. This practice supports the child's and family's overall development and respects their unique preferences and needs.

In children's play and activities, we must understand the importance of sensory-motor development. Motor skills involve intentional actions, along with planning and sequencing movements, which demand perception and attention. Autistic individuals often experience challenges related to motor skills. When we overlook individual differences—such as each child's sensory-motor profile—we may fail to see why a child struggles to sit properly, whether due to posture difficulties or vestibular issues. Likewise, challenges with motor planning can disrupt the organization of certain movements.

Direct physical manipulation to prompt a child to perform actions is a common practice aimed at ensuring children imitate or complete activities. This requires attention because it disturbs the child's bodily autonomy. The adult compels the child to follow the adult's schedule and desires and disregards the child's own intentions. If an adult compels a child to act, who is acting—the adult who issues commands or the child?

Each person's expressions, movements, and actions reveal their uniqueness. They reflect a bodily presence in the world, where sensory-motor aspects form a unified experience connected with language. Any respectful, sensitive approach must recognize the uniqueness of autistic individuals as essential—especially their sense of time.

Adjust communication timing and pacing to match the individual's rhythm when interacting with autistic individuals, promoting authentic and meaningful exchanges.

Another important point is that some people physically adjust an autistic child's face to encourage eye contact, even when the child has difficulty doing so naturally. This invasive action, which disregards the child's own pace, objectifies them. Why is this practice accepted for autistic children but not for non-autistic ones?

When someone calls out to a child, several steps occur before the gaze can be shared:

1. The child must first register the sound, determine its direction, and find it interesting.
2. They need to organize their body to move toward the sound they heard.

3. They must coordinate and sequence muscle movements to align with the intended direction.
4. Finally, they need to look at the person who emitted the sound and locate their face in space.

Even simple actions involve many factors, such as sensory-motor skills, timing, and unique communication traits. It's important to always respect the child's body and space. We need to understand the complexity of these interactions and honor their autonomy and dignity.

During evaluations of children who received behavioral interventions, we observed difficulty in initiating actions. Due to highly structured environments, these children often struggle to start actions independently. In the DIR model's praxis stages—Initiation, Planning, Sequencing, Execution, and Adaptation—the first stage, initiation, is often compromised. Approaches that don't consider the child's interests and intentions can negatively impact their development.

Today, most professionals and families prioritize discipline, with many pushing for very strict disciplinary actions, even for infants and young children. Reward-punishment approaches that simplify addressing children's complex emotions, feelings, and behaviors are backward and often harsh. Such methods can result in negativity, rebellion, fear, anxiety, trauma, and passivity. **Why opt for an impersonal caregiving method that could harm a child's healthy development?** Respecting their individuality and fostering their autonomy is crucial for promoting growth in a supportive and empathetic environment.

If a child becomes dysregulated, we should recognize that they might be losing control due to sensory overload, emotional distress, frustration, or discomfort they can't express. In such situations, the child needs help to regain composure. Instead of ignoring their behavior, we should offer comfort and be emotionally available to help them co-regulate.

This involves coming down to the child's level, sitting face-to-face with them, and ensuring they feel that their discomfort is understood and that they are supported in their distress. Acting coldly or ignoring the child should not be an option, as it creates emotional distance and undermines the opportunity for connection and reassurance. Offering empathetic and compassionate care in such moments is essential for fostering trust and helping the child recover their sense of equilibrium.

Sensations, for example, intensify in connection with the development of perception processes directed toward a target. This is why they can be actively cultivated in a child, but such cultivation should not be limited to simple and mechanical training of sensations through formal exercises. If I want to communicate to someone that I am feeling hot, I can express this through various expressive movements.

However, true understanding and communication only occur when I can place the sensation of heat I experienced within a category that my interlocutor recognizes. The word typically becomes available once the concept is ready. We begin to understand the effective relationship between a child's cognitive development and their social development when we recognize the unity between communication and generalization.

The behavioral perspective uses strategies and techniques proven by science. However, some of its origins raise ethical questions. Lovaas, who developed interventions for autistic children, first studied conversion therapy for homosexual people (Rekers & Lovaas, 1974). Also, using food as a reward, which was common in early studies and still happens sometimes, is ethically questionable today. So, just because something is scientifically proven doesn't mean we shouldn't review it to make sure it's ethical and respects human rights.

Many people have criticized controversial parts of behavioral intervention. Because of this, new approaches like "Humanized ABA", "Naturalistic ABA", and "Naturalistic Developmental Behavioral Intervention (NDBI)" are appearing. These try to fix the problems of traditional ABA by focusing on learning in natural settings.

This raises some questions. If we need to use the word 'humanized', does that mean it wasn't humanized before? Where did this practice come from? Why do we need this concept now?

We have already talked about how all knowledge comes from certain beliefs and ways of understanding the world. A theory's actions and ideas are shaped by those beliefs. So, asking questions like "How does this new approach view the individual?" or "Which theorists influenced its development?" help us understand its foundation. These questions show the true principles behind its practices and how it understands real-life experiences.

5. Final Considerations

Autism is a neurodevelopmental condition that affects social interaction, communication, behavior, sensory experiences, and motor skills in diverse ways. Recognizing that each neurodivergent individual develops along unique paths, distinct from typical patterns, is essential. When focus shifts to deficits, diagnoses, or perceived shortcomings, it fosters labeling, marginalization, and stigma, reducing the individual to their diagnosis. Families, psychologists, therapists, teachers, and society must acknowledge autism as an integral part of a person's identity. The priority should be understanding the individual's unique traits and potential, rather than the diagnosis alone.

Corporeality, affect, and language are inseparable dimensions of human experience. Ignoring these aspects in discussions about learning and development oversimplifies the complexity of teaching, learning, and the broader fields of psychology and education. Approaches focused only on behavior fail to capture the full depth of these processes.

Our relationship with the world is always constructed through corporeality, and our perception of it occurs in an integrated manner through a complex interaction between the body and the environment. This perspective underscores the notion that autism is not merely behavior. The autism spectrum encompasses a wide range of possibilities across sensory, motor, interactive, communicational, emotional, and behavioral aspects of development. Ignoring subjectivity risks the mistake of assuming that all individuals with the same diagnosis are alike.

The consulted literature and the historical and cultural context of practices with autistic individuals reveal the significant prominence of behavioral approaches and exclusionary practices. However, education is far more than behavior training. Autistic individuals are not merely passive recipients of content who must learn neurotypical behaviors to conform to societal expectations. In some practices that view autistic individuals in this way, under the gaze of others, learners are often objectified and not recognized as individuals.

This reductionist practice overlooks the richness of lived experience and human subjectivity. Instead, it is essential to recognize that autistic individuals actively construct meaning and knowledge. A holistic approach is necessary, viewing the body not as a mere machine but as the foundation of perception and understanding of the world. Additionally, relationships are the cornerstone of the learning process.

Traditional approaches, rooted in a reductionist perspective, overlook the complexity of bodily experience intertwined with subjectivity by focusing solely on behavior. This narrow focus limits the understanding of autistic individuals' experiences, relying on superficial and fragmented analyses of their interaction with the world.

Inclusion is fundamentally connected to individuality. Health and education professionals must be trained to drive transformation, value differences, and act as agents of change. Strengthening partnerships between the health and education sectors and fostering collaborative initiatives and training to address gaps in supporting autistic individuals are essential steps forward.

All human beings are different, but in the context of ASD, there are unique traits that professionals must acknowledge, respect, study, and address with sensitivity. This approach prevents exclusion and supports autistic individuals by creating pathways of communication that promote their learning and development. Every autistic individual is unique.

To transform therapeutic and educational practices, we must create environments that respect individual uniqueness. These spaces should encourage meaningful dialogue, draw from lived experiences, prioritize intersubjective relationships, and align with the coexistence and interests of autistic individuals. The focus should shift to abilities rather than vulnerabilities, viewing autistic individuals as learners and providing conditions that enable their growth and success.

The current challenges lie in fostering a revolution in how we view and perceive each autistic individual with sensitivity. This calls for a shift in how we interact and the development of new therapeutic and educational practices. These practices must respect each person's unique differences and recognize them as active participants in the process of building their own knowledge. It requires focusing on the affective and relational aspects of learning, shifting from traditional views to embracing differences as a path to humanization and belonging.

These changes are urgent and must happen with clarity and purpose, understanding why change is necessary and approaching it thoughtfully. This intentional approach is essential for building a more inclusive and compassionate society that values diversity as a cornerstone of human connection and growth.

References

American Medical Association. (2023). *House of Delegates Annual Meeting, Resolution 706: Revision of H-185.921, Removal of AMA Support for Applied Behavior Analysis.* AMA House of Delegates Handbook, pp. 1179–1182.

American Psychiatric Association. (2013). *Diagnostic and Statistical Manual of Mental Disorders: DSM-5* (5th Edn.). Arlington, VA: American Psychiatric Publishing.

American Psychiatric Association. (2022). *Manual Diagnóstico e Estatístico de Transtornos Mentais: DSM-5-TR* (5th Edn., revised text). Porto Alegre: Artmed.

Araújo, A.M.L. de. (2023). *Estratégias musicais aplicadas ao modelo DIR/FLOORTIME: Possíveis contribuições para o desenvolvimento de crianças autistas* (Master's dissertation). Programa de Pós-Graduação em Humanidades, Instituto Federal do Espírito Santo, Vitória, Brazil.

Brazelton, T.B. and Greenspan, S. (2002). *As necessidades essenciais das crianças: O que cada criança precisa para crescer, aprender e se desenvolver.* Porto Alegre: Artes Médicas.

Bunge, M. (1980). *Epistemologia.* São Paulo: Queiroz Editor.

Casenhiser, D. M., Shanker, S. and Stieben, J. (2011). Learning through interaction in children with autism: Preliminary data from a social-communication-based intervention. *Autism, 15*(2), 123–146. https://doi.org/10.1177/1362361311422052.

Christian, G. (2011). A person-centered approach to problem behavior: Using DIR®/ Floortime with adults who have severe developmental delays. *Autism Advocate, 14*(2), 21–31. Bethesda, MD: Autism Society.

Greenspan, S. (1993). *Entrevista clínica com crianças* (2nd Edn.). Porto Alegre: Artes Médicas.

Greenspan, S. (2000). *Filhos emocionalmente saudáveis, íntegros, felizes, inteligentes.* Rio de Janeiro: Campus.

Greenspan, S. and Wieder, S. (2006). *Engaging Autism: Using the Floortime Approach to Help Children Relate, Communicate, and Think.* Da Capo Press.

Lal, R. and Chhabria, R. (2013). Early intervention of autism: A case for Floor Time approach. In: *Recent Advances in Autism Spectrum Disorders I.* https://doi.org/10.5772/54378.

Lampreia, C. (2007). A perspectiva desenvolvimentista para intervenção precoce no autismo. *Estudos de Psicologia, 24*(1), 105–114.

Leal, A.R.G. (2018). *Modelo DIR/Floortime: Bases teóricas para a inclusão de crianças com autismo na educação infantil* (Master's dissertation). Universidade Federal do Piauí, Teresina, Brazil.

Orrú, S.E. (2016). *Aprendizes com autismo: Aprendizagem por eixos de interesse em espaços não excludentes.* Rio de Janeiro: Vozes.

Pajareya, K. and Kopmaneejumruslers, K. (2011). A pilot randomized controlled trial of DIR/Floortime™ parent training intervention for pre-school children with autistic spectrum disorders. *Autism, 15*(2), 1–15. https://doi.org/10.1177/1362361310386502.

Pajareya, K., Sutchritpongs, S. and Kongkasuwan, R. (2019). DIR/Floortime® parent training intervention for children with developmental disabilities: A randomized controlled trial. *Siriraj Medical Journal, 71*(5), 331–338.

Papalia, D.E. and Martorelli, G. (2022). *Desenvolvimento humano* (14th Edn.). Porto Alegre: Artmed.

Rekers, G.A. and Lovaas, O.I. (1974). Behavioral treatment of deviant sex-role behaviors in a male child. *Journal of Applied Behavior Analysis, 7*(2), 173–190. https://doi.org/10.1901/jaba.1974.7-173.

Sandbank, M., Bottema-Beutel, K., Crowley, S., Cassidy, M., Dunham, K., Feldman, J.I., Crank, J., Albarran, S.A., Raj, S., Mahbub, P. and Woynaroski, T.G. (2020). Project AIM: Autism intervention meta-analysis for studies of young children. *Psychological Bulletin, 146*(1), 1–29. https://doi.org/10.1037/bul0000215.

Solomon, R. (2013). O Projeto Play: Um modelo de treinamento de formadores de intervenção precoce para crianças com transtornos do espectro do autismo. In: C. Schmidt (Ed.), *Autismo, educação e transdisciplinaridade* (pp. xx–xx). Campinas: Papirus.

Solomon, R., Van Egeren, L., Mahoney, G., Quon Huber, M. and Zimmerman, P. (2014). PLAY Project Home Consultation Intervention Program for Young Children with Autism Spectrum Disorders: A randomized controlled trial. *Journal of Developmental and Behavioral Pediatrics, 35*(8), 475–485. https://doi.org/10.1097/DBP.0000000000000096.

Vygotsky, L.S. (2007). *A formação social da mente: O desenvolvimento dos processos psicológicos superiores* (7th Edn.). São Paulo: Martins Fontes.

5 Advanced Strategies for ASD Detection
A Narrative Review

Adrielly Sayonara[1*], Camila Narjara[1], Thailson[1],
Maria Euclécia A. da Silva[1], Juliana C. Gomes Cassemiro[1] and
Wellington Pinheiro dos Santos[1]

This chapter presents a narrative review of methodologies that researchers use in multiple studies to achieve early diagnosis of Autism Spectrum Disorder (ASD) with electroencephalographic (EEG) signals and machine learning. EEG emerges as a promising tool to identify patterns linked to ASD. Researchers combine it with advanced preprocessing techniques and machine learning algorithms. The text first highlights brain patterns revealed by EEG. Then it describes preprocessing approaches, such as band-pass filtering, windowing, the Fourier Transform, and Independent Component Analysis (ICA). Additional techniques, such as the Short-Time Fourier Transform (STFT) and wavelet transforms, capture temporal and frequency features. The chapter then explores classifiers, including neural networks and support vector machines (SVM). Researchers select these methods based on data characteristics and study goals. This choice aims to optimize diagnostic accuracy. Combining different approaches strengthens model robustness. The final section addresses the limitations of these methods. These constraints involve reliance on multimodal data, high computational complexity, and the specificity of frequency bands and EEG channels. Despite these challenges, advancements in EEG and machine learning for ASD diagnosis offer immense potential. They can reshape diagnostics and improve the quality of life for affected individuals.

1. Introduction

Autism Spectrum Disorder (ASD) is a neuropsychiatric condition that profoundly affects social, communicative, and behavioral development from the first few years of life. Researchers detect ASD signs within the first 12 months (Maestro et al., 2005). The disorder shows broad and variable manifestations. It includes restricted social interactions, impaired nonverbal

1 Federal University of Pernambuco, Recife, Brazil.
* Corresponding author: adrielly.sayonara@ufpe.br

DOI: 10.1201/9781003531418-5

communication, and repetitive behavior patterns. These characteristics create a unique experience for individuals with ASD. Early diagnosis and personalized intervention strategies foster better development and social integration (Napolitano et al., 2022).

Public awareness of ASD has grown significantly in recent decades. However, many challenges persist in early identification and in the implementation of effective interventions. Researchers must develop diagnostic methods that detect ASD in its initial stages. This approach accelerates specialized therapies and improves outcomes for individuals within this spectrum.

Many recent studies (Radhakrishnan et al., 2021; Sanabria-Barradas et al., 2022; Wadhera et al., 2023) use electroencephalogram (EEG) and artificial intelligence (AI) to find early diagnostic methods for ASD. Researchers explore specific patterns of brain activity related to ASD. This approach enables more precise and agile detection of the condition in early development. They combine EEG data with AI algorithms and create diagnostic tools that are more sensitive and specific. They also aim for accessibility and noninvasive procedures.

This chapter evaluates the use of AI techniques in the analysis of EEG data for early ASD diagnosis. The objective is to identify the most commonly employed techniques and the challenges in their implementation. The text also examines possible applications, limitations, and future development opportunities.

For this chapter, the authors conducted a narrative review of publications from 2019 to 2024. They selected articles on the Semantic Scholar platform, focusing on academically relevant research published in prominent journals and scientific events. They prioritized works that address the use of EEG signals and AI techniques in ASD diagnosis. This selection includes significant and methodologically robust contributions in the field.

2. Main Investigations

2.1 EEG and ASD Databases

The nineteen articles in this chapter rely on multiple EEG databases. Some authors make these databases publicly available. They differ in the number of participants, electrode configurations, sampling rates, data collection protocols, and demographic or clinical characteristics. This variety reflects different approaches and contexts in ASD diagnosis research with EEG signals and AI. Most databases come from clinical settings. They contain neurotypical individuals and individuals with ASD, with ages from childhood to adulthood. Table 1 details each database in the selected studies.

Three studies (Melinda et al., 2023; Mohi-ud Din and Jayanthy, 2021; Tawhid et al., 2021) use a dataset from King Abdulaziz University. That dataset includes only 18 participants. Other works (Ali et al., 2022; Mohi-ud Din and Jayanthy, 2023) rely on data from the Simons Foundation for Autism Research Initiative (SFARI). The largest datasets appear in the studies by Baygin et al. (2021) and Abdulhay et al. (2022). They include 122 volunteers: 61 neurotypical individuals and 61 with ASD.

2.2 Brain Patterns and Features Found through EEG

Children with ASD have a higher density of neuronal connections than neurotypical children. A reduction in the natural neuronal pruning process causes this change. Pruning eliminates damaged neurons during brain development (Oh et al., 2021). This increased connectivity leads to a non-uniform pattern of brain activation. Children with ASD show a lack of synchronization among cognitive functions in different brain regions and a pronounced disconnection, especially between frontal and posterior areas. These observations indicate a brain with more numerous neural connections (Oh et al., 2021).

Magnetic resonance imaging (MRI) and computed tomography (CT) studies reveal a larger brain size in children with ASD, most prominently in the temporal and frontal lobes. However, the specialists do not recommend these imaging techniques for ASD diagnosis because they do not correlate consistently with clinical symptoms. Moreover, children with ASD often need sedation for these exams. Enclosed machines and the need to remain still cause discomfort, which presents challenges. CT also exposes patients to ionizing radiation, and MRI entails high costs and limited availability (Baygin et al., 2021). EEG offers a promising diagnostic alternative. It has low cost, portability, ease of use, and a noninvasive, painless procedure (Ieracitano et al., 2019).

EEG measures brain activity over time. It records voltage changes from ionic current flow among neurons. Researchers place electrodes on the scalp in standardized positions, often under the 10–20 or 10–10 international systems. A conductive paste holds the electrodes in position and improves conduction. This setup lowers unwanted capacitance or resistance from movement or hair.

EEG signals range from 0 to 300 μV, with frequencies from 0.5 to 100 Hz in typical conditions. Brain rhythms depend on many factors and vary widely. In alert states, neurons desynchronize and generate lower amplitude, higher frequency signals. In relaxed states, neurons synchronize and produce greater amplitude, lower frequency signals. Frequency bands include delta (0.5–4 Hz), theta (4–8 Hz), alpha (8–13 Hz), beta (13–32 Hz), and gamma (32–100 Hz).

Table 1 Description of the databases used by the articles in the narrative review presented in this chapter

Author(s)	*Signals*	*Electrode System*	*Number of Electroders*	*Database*	*Number of participants*	*Sampling frequency*
Baygin et al. (2021)	EEG	10-20	64	Own	122(61 ASD, 61 TD)	500 Hz
De Oliveira Silva et al. (2024)	EEG	10-10	9 (FT7, FC5, FC3, FC1, FCz, FC2, FC4 FC6 and FT8)	Sheffield	56(28 ASD, 28TD)	512 Hz
Han et al. (2022)	EEG and Eye-tracking	*	128	Own	90(40 ASD, 50 TD)	1000 Hz (EEG Datal) 300 Hz (ET Data)
Tasnim et al. (2022)	EEG	*	8(C3, Cz, C4, CPz, P3, P4, POz, Pz)	BCIAUT-P300	15	250 Hz
Melinda et al. (2023)	EEG	10-20	16(FP1, F3, F7, T3, T5, O1, C4, FP2, FZ, F4, F8, C3, CZ, PZ, OZ AND O2)	King Abdulaziz University (UKA)	18(8 ASD, 10 TD)	256 Hz
Radhakrishnan et al. (2022)	EEG	10-20	19(Fp1, Fp2, F7, F3, Fz, F4, F8, P3, P4, Pz, T3, T5, T4, T6)	Own	*	500 Hz
Chen et al. (2023)	EEG	10-20	32	A total of 29 databases downloaded by openneuro	4899	250 Hz
Rechal et al. (2021)	EEG	*	8(C3, Cz, C4, CPz, P3, P4, POz, Pz)	BCIAUT-P300	15	250 Hz
Oh et al. (2021)	EEG	10-20	64	Own	77(40 ASD, 37 TD)	500 Hz
Tawhid et al. (2021)	EEG	10-20	16(F7, Fp1, Fp2, F8, F3, Fz, F4, T3, C3, Cz C4, T5, O1, Oz, O2, Pz)	King Abdulaziz University (KAU)	16(12 ASD. 4 TD)	256 Hz

Contd.

Table 1 *Contd.*

Author(s)	*Signals*	*Electrode System*	*Number of Electroders*	*Database*	*Number of participants*	*Sampling frequency*
Wadhera et al. (2023)	EEG	10-20	32	Dataset I - King Abdulaziz University (KAU), Dataset II and III - Own	63 (50 ASD, 13 TD)	256 Hz
Mohi-ud Din and Jayanthy (2023)	EEG	10-20	128	Simons Foundation for Autism Research Initiative (SFARI)	28 (14 ASD, 14 TD)	500 Hz
Kansara et al. (2024)	EEG	10-20	14	Physionet	5	*
Ali et al. (2022)	EEG	10-20	128	Simons Foundation for Autism Research Initiative (SFARI) and Database Boston Children's	53(38 ASD, 14 TD)	500 Hz
Abdulhav et al. (2022)	EEG	10-20	64	*	122 (61 ASD, 61 TD)	500 Hz
Menaka et al. (2023)	EEG	10-20	8 (O1, O2, T7, T8, F4, F3, F7, and F8)	Own	20(10 ASD, 10 TD)	*
Peng et al. (2021)	EEG	10-20	14(AF3, F7, F3, FC5, T7, P7, O1, O2, P8, T8, FC6, F4, F8, and)	Own	80	*
Mohi-ud Din and Jayanthy (2021)	EEG	10-20	16	King Abdulaziz University (KAU)	17(13 ASD, 4 TD)	256 Hz
Jayawardana et al. (2019)	EEG	10-20	32	Own	52(24 ASD, 28 TD)	250 Hz

Researchers analyze EEG signals to identify neurological diseases. Excessive or uncontrolled brain activity, slowed rhythms, or altered synchronization may indicate neural dysfunction or degeneration. Clinicians use EEG to diagnose epilepsy (Tatum et al., 2018), Alzheimer's disease (Bairagi and Elgandelwar, 2023), and brain injuries from tumors or strokes (Tong et al., 2024). This technique also assists in evaluating sleep disorders (Peter-Derex et al., 2021).

Oh et al. (2021) and Baygin et al. (2021) propose automatic ASD detection systems with EEG signals and machine learning algorithms. Both studies use 64 channels to record EEG from children aged 4–13 years. Oh et al. study 40 children with ASD and 37 without atypical development. They collect signals at a 500 Hz sampling rate and focus on a 0.3–40 Hz frequency range. They extract 18 nonlinear and explicit attributes, most of which center on entropy, because entropy describes signal complexity across multiple time scales (Han et al., 2022). They then select, reduce, and rank the best attributes with Student's t-test and Marginal Fisher Analysis. They use the three most significant attributes to develop an autism index.

Baygin et al. (2021) study 122 subjects, equally split between ASD and controls, covering mild, moderate, and severe ASD. They propose a method that converts brain signals into spectrograms and applies hybrid deep architectures. Pre-trained deep networks extract the attributes, and shallow classifiers operate in the final layer.

Han et al. (2022) also adopt a high-electrode density method for EEG data collection. They include 90 children, with 40 who have ASD and 50 who exhibit typical development, between 3 and 6 years old. They place 128 electrodes on each child's scalp and collect signals at 1000 Hz for at least a few minutes. They focus on 62 electrodes for the analysis. These cover frontal, central, temporal, occipital, and parietal regions in both hemispheres. They extract features from multiple domains, emphasizing power features due to evidence that resting EEG in autistic children shows reduced alpha power and increased power in delta and theta bands. They compute power in each channel and then average it in each frequency band. They also extract entropy-based features and connectivity metrics.

Many studies report promising results in automatic autism detection. However, systems with many electrodes do not offer a practical approach. High-density EEG systems are not common in clinical settings. Smaller configurations may also benefit autistic children by reducing discomfort during data collection. Researchers must identify which brain regions are more strongly affected. This knowledge would allow the use of fewer electrodes while maintaining diagnostic accuracy.

Melinda et al. (2023) evaluated 16 children, including eight with ASD. They used 16 electrodes at FP1, F3, F7, T3, T5, O1, C4, FP2, FZ, F4, F8, C3, CZ, PZ, and O2 (reference). The analysis focused on the beta frequency range and reached an accuracy of up to 99%. This work provides an initial view, but the sample remains limited.

Radhakrishnan et al. (2022) compared brain signals from six children, three with ASD and three with typical development. They placed 19 electrodes according to the 10-20 system at Fp1, Fp2, F7, F3, Fz, F4, F8, P3, P4, Pz, T3, T5, T4, T6, O1, O2, C3, C4, and Cz. They applied three anomaly-detection models with PyCaret. Anomalies are events or observations that deviate significantly from the rest of the data. The Angle-based Outlier Detector identified T5, Fp2, and Pz as anomalous in children with ASD. The Isolation Forest model flagged Pz for all ASD children. The Minimum Covariance Determinant model indicated Fp2, Pz, and P3. These results suggest that the frontoparietal regions may serve as key indicators for ASD diagnosis via EEG.

Other researchers also investigated low-density EEG. Peng et al. (2021) and Kansara et al. (2024) used the EMOTIV EPOC+ system. This portable, high-resolution device features 14 electrodes at AF3, F7, F3, FC5, T7, P7, O1, O2, P8, T8, FC6, F4, F8, and AF4, plus two references (P3 and P4). Signals transfer wirelessly through Bluetooth. Peng et al. (2021) recruited 64 children aged 4 to 6. Instead of resting-state signals, they chose event-related potentials (ERPs) while presenting positive and negative emotional stimuli.

ERP is a specific type of brain signal. It influences cognitive processes such as information processing, working memory, and intelligence. The study's methodology involved splitting the different frequency bands and extracting 20 features. These include time-based and frequency-based features. The authors observed that, under positive emotional stimuli, the beta rhythm provides better discrimination, followed by the alpha rhythm.

Under negative emotional stimuli, the theta rhythm shows the strongest discrimination. The authors also analyzed how different brain regions affect signal differentiation. Contrary to previous findings, they noted that features from the occipital lobe offer the highest classification accuracy under emotional stimuli. This effect may connect to visual processing in the occipital lobe, given that the study employed videos during EEG data collection.

Menaka et al. (2024) then achieved approximately 90% accuracy when distinguishing between children with ASD and those with typical development. The study involved 20 participants, evenly split between the two groups, ages 5–7 years. It used only eight electrodes, placed on the occipital, central, and temporal lobes at O1, O2, T7, T8, F4, F3, F7, and F8. Like Peng et al. (2021), the authors presented a video stimulus. This approach provided insights into each child's concentration level during the stimulus.

Different studies do not show a clear consensus on which brain regions display the most activation and effectively separate autistic children from nonautistic children. Several investigations indicate that 8–14 electrodes may suffice. This finding highlights the feasibility of simpler EEG systems. These simpler systems become more accessible and better suited for the target audience. Researchers should direct future investigations toward this approach.

2.3 Application of Artificial Intelligence Techniques in EEG Analysis

Computational neuroscience holds a key role in research involving AI for EEG analysis. These methods enable brain mapping and support early ASD diagnosis. This section discusses preprocessing techniques and recurrent classifiers, as the literature describes.

2.3.1 Preprocessing Techniques

Preprocessing EEG signals removes unwanted noise and artifacts. It improves the signal-to-noise ratio and segments the signal into specific intervals, such as time windows. This approach facilitates the analysis of certain temporal events or patterns. Standardizing the amplitude also helps compare different data segments or individuals. These steps enhance subsequent analyses that extract information from EEG signals through AI.

Many researchers combine more than one preprocessing technique to optimize EEG signal quality. Han et al. (2022) applied both band-pass filtering and windowing. Band-pass filtering is widespread. It removes noise and artifacts irrelevant to brain signal analysis. Ali et al. (2022), Menaka et al. (2024), Han et al. (2022), and Mohi-ud Din and Jayanthy (2021) underscore the importance of band-pass filtering. It eliminates artifacts from eye movements (EOG) and electrical networks, retaining only essential frequencies for analysis.

It is essential to set careful criteria when choosing the frequency band and filter characteristics. This approach avoids discarding relevant information in the signal. Filters with abrupt transitions can distort signals in the time domain. Poorly defined frequency bands can suppress neural components that matter for certain analyses. The selection of an ideal frequency band aligns with the neurophysiological phenomenon under study. It considers the frequency bands associated with brain activities of interest, such as delta, theta, alpha, beta, or gamma.

Windowing segments EEG signals over time. This method reveals detailed temporal variations in the signals. Combining these preprocessing techniques enhances data quality and strengthens feature extraction and classification.

This integrated approach supports more accurate and robust machine learning models. It improves the ability to detect ASD-related patterns, raising diagnostic accuracy and reliability.

Like Han et al. (2022), Peng et al. (2021) also used windowing, with a 4-second window and a 2-second overlap. This overlapping window method ensures continuous capture of temporal transitions in the signals. It produces a more faithful representation of EEG data.

Baygin et al. (2021) applied the Fourier Transform to analyze EEG signals across frequency and time. This approach handles non-stationary signals more precisely. The transform's linearity converts a linear combination of signals into a linear combination of their transforms and allows time shifting. This decomposition of EEG signals into frequency components helps identify relevant patterns.

Furthermore, the authors implement a feature generation technique called 1D Local Binary Pattern (1D LBP). This method relies on nine-dimensional microstructures to produce features. In practice, 1D LBP inspects small signal windows and generates a binary pattern for each point based on its neighbors. This process creates a feature vector of length 256. It captures local variations in EEG signals and uncovers subtle details, which support robust machine learning models for ASD detection and classification.

Eye blinks and muscle movements corrupt EEG signals with noise that obscures real brain activity patterns. Researchers often use advanced methods such as Independent Component Analysis (ICA) to reduce these effects. ICA applies statistical techniques that separate mixed signals into independent components. This strategy identifies and isolates distinct artifacts.

Studies by Kansara et al. (2024), Peng et al. (2021), Melinda et al. (2023), Wadhera et al. (2023), and Jayawardana et al. (2019) highlight the effectiveness of ICA in EEG preprocessing. These authors use ICA to remove artifacts and reveal genuine brain activity patterns. Thorough artifact removal enhances EEG signal quality and boosts performance in subsequent feature extraction and classification.

Wavelet transforms also serve as advanced preprocessing approaches. They decompose signals into multiple frequencies and note the exact moments when these frequencies appear. This technique presents a combined temporal and frequency perspective. It exposes variations in signal segments at different scales and resolutions.

Wavelet transforms include different subtypes. Each subtype has distinct traits and specific uses. The Continuous Wavelet Transform (CWT) produces a continuous, detailed representation of the signal in frequency and time domains. Researchers rely on it to detect subtle, complex patterns.

Chen et al. (2023) used CWT to extract EEG features. The Discrete Wavelet Transform (DWT) provides multi-resolution analysis. This method compresses EEG signals and detects distinct events at various time scales. Melinda et al. (2023) applied DWT to segment and compress EEG data without losing critical details. Both the continuous and discrete wavelets transform the refined EEG signals. They offer local analysis at different scales and resolutions, as shown in recent studies (Mohi-ud Din and Jayanthy, 2021).

Rechal et al. (2021) presented an autism detection algorithm based on EEG signal processing. The authors applied Variational Mode Decomposition (VMD) in the preprocessing step. VMD breaks down EEG signals into distinct components. It adapts to each signal's characteristics and aligns with its variations.

VMD uses a variational search method to optimize decomposition. This approach identifies a set of modes that accurately represent the original signal. Each mode covers a frequency band with specific properties, revealing multiple signal aspects. This adaptability benefits complex signals such as EEG.

VMD enables a more detailed EEG signal analysis. It uncovers patterns and variations hidden in broad analyses. Its ability to isolate key components and reduce noise or artifacts improves clarity. This feature makes VMD a powerful technique for EEG data preprocessing.

This level of adaptive decomposition is crucial. It extracts relevant features from EEG signals and supports early ASD detection. VMD segments signals and uncovers detailed brain activity. This approach improves the accuracy and reliability of machine learning models for ASD classification and diagnosis (Rechal et al., 2021).

Researchers often use the T-test for feature selection in data preparation. This statistical test compares mean differences between two groups. It identifies the most discriminative features, removes noise, and excludes irrelevant values. These steps enhance model performance.

The T-test directs the analysis toward key features. It increases accuracy and efficiency, especially for complex signals like EEG. This approach pinpoints the most significant information and mitigates noise or variability unrelated to brain activity. Oh et al. (2021) exemplify T-test usage in EEG data preparation. They remove irrelevant features and highlight crucial ones. This procedure produces a more robust model. Oh et al. (2021) also apply Multiple Factor Analysis (MFA) to EEG signals. They address datasets with diverse characteristics. MFA reduces dimensionality and adapts to intricate data with varied features.

MFA locates and extracts the most relevant variables. It simplifies data structure and improves interpretation of underlying patterns. This approach reduces dimensionality, increases computational efficiency, and boosts the accuracy of later analysis models. It selects more specific and relevant attributes, removes noise and redundancy, and supports robust analyses. This method clarifies EEG data and enables focused, effective investigations that detect important features.

In the study by Tasnim et al. (2022), the dataset showed an imbalance between ASD and non-ASD classes. The authors used data augmentation to fix this imbalance and enhance model generalization. Data augmentation creates new data from the original set, increases model generalization, and reduces overfitting.

One popular technique is the Synthetic Minority Over-sampling Technique (SMOTE). It generates synthetic samples of the minority class, rather than duplicating the existing ones. This strategy selects minority-class samples, combines them to form new examples, and balances the class distribution. A balanced dataset leads to improved performance, making models more robust and accurate. However, the test set should include only the original data.

As previously stated, noise and artifacts often degrade EEG signals. Researchers use effective preprocessing techniques to ensure clarity and usefulness. Tawhid et al. (2021) describe Common Average Referencing (CAR). This method computes the average of all electrodes and subtracts that average from each electrode's value. It reduces noise common to all electrodes while highlighting each electrode's specific variations. CAR's computational simplicity makes it popular for EEG preprocessing. It improves the signal-to-noise ratio and clarifies the data for interpretation.

Some datasets require value adjustments. Normalization is essential for scaling variables, supporting accurate comparisons among them. It prevents certain features from dominating due to differing scales. This step boosts analysis accuracy, especially when data integrity is critical. Tawhid et al. (2021) and Abdulhay et al. (2022) illustrate the effectiveness of normalization in preparing data for advanced analysis. Proper normalization strengthens preprocessing and ensures that machine learning models operate with maximum efficiency, producing robust and generalizable results.

Some datasets lack information about certain electrodes. de Oliveira Silva et al. (2024) address this gap by imputing missing values and preserving data integrity. They apply Inverse Distance Weighting (IDW), which calculates a weighted average of nearby electrodes. It assigns higher weight to closer electrodes and less weight to those farther away. This technique, originally used in geostatistics, fits EEG data well because signals are spatially arranged on the scalp. It delivers more accurate estimates for missing values.

Preprocessing EEG signals is crucial for early ASD diagnosis. The techniques in this chapter improve data quality and reveal relevant features.

Each method offers specific advantages, depending on the data and the study objectives. Proper application uncovers essential information from EEG signals. This approach supports research and clinical practice in computational neuroscience.

2.3.2 *Classifiers*

Classifiers are algorithms that categorize datasets with distinct characteristics. They recognize patterns and attributes in data and then assign categories to different classes. These algorithms organize relevant information and ensure that new examples fit the categories based on previously learned features. In early ASD diagnosis, researchers use a range of classifiers, from simple to sophisticated. They rely on mathematical foundations such as linear algebra, probability, statistics, calculus, and information theory. These concepts guide accurate data analysis and decision-making for categorizing new examples.

Artificial neural networks, inspired by the human brain, are advanced computational models that learn and detect complex patterns. They consist of interconnected "artificial neurons", which process information in a way reminiscent of biological neural networks. In the context of ASD, they excel at detecting specific patterns in complex data, such as EEG signals, and provide novel diagnostic support. The literature reveals many methods and architectures for neural networks. Their inherent flexibility accommodates configurations such as convolutional, recurrent, or fully connected layers. Researchers also use regularization, optimization, and hyperparameter tuning to adapt these models to tasks like time series analysis or nonlinear feature detection.

Neural networks show promising results for ASD diagnosis. Recent studies, such as Rechal et al. (2021), report accuracy as high as 97.08%. These findings highlight the potential of neural networks to transform complex signals into precise clinical indicators. This progress broadens the reach of AI in neuroscience and paves the way for more personalized and effective diagnostic approaches.

In the study by Tasnim et al. (2022), the Multi-Layer Perceptron (MLP) produced limited results, reaching only 56.42% accuracy. MLP is a classic neural network architecture with multiple interconnected layers of neurons. These hidden layers learn and transform data representations. Although MLP can model complex relationships, its structural simplicity restricts certain applications. One main limitation is its inability to capture temporal or sequential dependencies, which are central in EEG analysis. MLP processes the signal statically, overlooking correlations between different time points. This characteristic undermines its effectiveness for tasks that need deeper temporal insights. MLP also risks overfitting, especially with high-dimensional or small datasets, which are common in neuroscience. Hyperparameter tuning can help, but requires expertise and does not ensure robust results. These factors justify the use of more specialized networks, such as recurrent or convolutional architectures, which handle temporal signals more effectively.

Forward Neural Networks (FNNs) process information in one direction, with no cycles or feedback. These networks may include one or more hidden layers, where adjustable weights and biases transform inputs into more abstract representations. This unidirectional path converts raw data into information useful for decisions or predictions. Although FNNs are widely effective, their static nature makes them less ideal for tasks involving temporal or sequential data. In these contexts, architectures like Recurrent Neural Networks (RNNs), Gated Recurrent Units (GRUs), or Long Short-Term Memory (LSTMs) handle temporal relationships more effectively. Still, Mohi ud Din and Jayanthy (2023) report an 88% accuracy with an FNN, showing its competence in problems that do not require complex temporal processing. This result confirms the adaptability of FNNs in scenarios where static features suffice, reinforcing their importance in specific artificial intelligence applications.

Convolutional Neural Networks (CNNs) are a specialized form of Artificial Neural Network. They handle data with spatial or temporal structure, such as images or EEG signals. Traditional Neural Networks rely on fully connected layers, where each neuron connects to all neurons in the next layer. CNNs instead use convolutional layers. These layers apply filters (or kernels) to detect local patterns in the data. After the convolutional steps, CNNs use pooling layers. This technique reduces dimensionality and keeps the most relevant features. It enables tasks such as pattern recognition and classification. CNNs learn hierarchical representations of the data and capture complex spatial and temporal patterns. They are effective in processing images, EEG signals, and other structured data (Chen et al., 2023; Kansara et al., 2024; Tawhid et al., 2021). Tawhid et al. (2021) tested various CNN models and attained 99.15% accuracy, demonstrating significant performance.

AlexNet is a recognized CNN architecture. It has 8 layers, with 5 convolutional layers that use kernels to detect specific patterns in the input. The network then includes 3 fully connected layers. Each neuron in these layers connects to every neuron in the previous layer. Between the convolutional and fully connected layers, pooling layers reduce feature map dimensionality and decrease computational demands. AlexNet also incorporates dropout layers. Dropout deactivates some neurons during training and promotes model generalization. This robust design allows AlexNet to learn hierarchical data features, making it very effective in complex pattern recognition tasks.

Menaka et al. (2024) reported an 85.16% accuracy for AlexNet in a pattern recognition task. The model handled large volumes of data efficiently. The authors then proposed an improved version of the model. They added extra convolutional layers, modified the optimizer, and adjusted the learning rate. These changes raised accuracy to 90.12%, showing that architectural tweaks and hyperparameter adjustments can further improve CNNs in demanding machine learning problems.

VGG16 is a deep CNN with 16 trainable layers, including 13 convolutional layers and 3 fully connected layers. This added depth extracts more complex and detailed features from input data. VGG16 is especially effective for EEG image and signal analysis. Its 3x3 filters capture subtle patterns in high-resolution data, while its final 3 fully connected layers consolidate the extracted features. This design supports advanced pattern recognition tasks. Researchers often use VGG16 in computer vision scenarios, including ASD detection and diagnosis. Menaka et al. (2024) report an accuracy of 50%, showing VGG16's capacity for large-scale, high-dimensional data. However, its depth demands caution to avoid overfitting, especially with limited data.

Menaka et al. (2024) also explored ResNet50, an advanced CNN with 50 layers: 48 convolutional layers, one max-pooling layer, and one average-pooling layer. ResNet50 achieved an accuracy of 75.15%. It uses residual connections, which carry information across layers instead of forcing a strict sequential path. This approach simplifies deep network training and alleviates gradient degradation. Residual connections enable richer representations and more effective detection of complex patterns. The depth of ResNet50, coupled with its residual connections, uncovers subtle, detailed features that are essential in diagnostic contexts. The pooling layers reduce data dimensionality and highlight key features without losing the complexity required for EEG analysis.

ResNet50 combines depth, efficient connectivity, and pooling techniques. It excels at diagnostic tasks with temporal and dynamic signals, including early ASD diagnosis.

SqueezeNet offers highly efficient CNN architecture. It reduces model size without sacrificing performance. It uses a "squeeze and expand" approach, shrinking and then expanding features. This design lowers model complexity while retaining essential information. It includes 18 convolutional layers that extract features and apply standard pooling to reduce dimensionality. Its compact structure eases storage demands and lowers computational costs. In the context of early ASD diagnosis, SqueezeNet processes scalograms derived from EEG signals, transforming temporal and frequency data into visual representations for convolutional layers. This method captures both temporal and spectral patterns, crucial for accurate data analysis. Mohi-ud Din and Jayanthy (2021) achieved about 83% accuracy with SqueezeNet, confirming its efficiency and robustness in complex biomedical signal analysis. Its strong performance and minimal resource needs make it ideal for portable and cost-effective scenarios where efficiency matters.

GoogLeNet, developed by Google in 2014, advances CNN architecture through Inception Modules. These modules process multiple convolution sizes (1 × 1, 3 × 3, and 5 × 5) and a 3 × 3 max pooling in parallel, then merge the results into a single layer. This design captures varied data features while reducing parameters, improving computational efficiency. GoogLeNet has 22 trainable layers (or 27 with pooling). It applies 1 × 1 convolutions for dimensionality reduction before the larger-scale convolutions, which lowers complexity. Instead of traditional fully connected layers, it uses global average pooling at the end, cutting parameter counts and boosting generalization. It also relies on auxiliary classifiers during training to prevent vanishing gradients, aiding deeper-layer learning. As a pre-trained model, GoogLeNet adapts to new tasks by leveraging knowledge from large datasets. Mohi-ud Din and Jayanthy (2021) report a 75% accuracy rate with GoogLeNet on EEG-based ASD diagnosis. Its blend of efficiency and high-level pattern recognition makes it a strategic option for early ASD detection and other medical applications that involve complex biomedical data.

RNNs handle sequential and temporal data. They maintain an internal state that reflects past information. This trait helps in analyzing EEG signals, which change over time and require the capture of temporal dependencies. RNNs detect complex patterns that show changes in brain activity, making them useful for ASD diagnosis. Wadhera et al. (2023) achieved an accuracy of 86.89% with RNNs.

LSTM extends RNNs to capture long-term dependencies found in time-series data like EEG signals. Traditional RNNs face the vanishing gradient problem. LSTMs resolve this with a gate mechanism that regulates information flow and preserves important memories. This feature is vital for identifying EEG patterns related to ASD. Bidirectional LSTMs (Bi-LSTMs) process data in both directions, enriching the temporal context and enhancing the detection of complex patterns. Wadhera et al. (2023) report 93.37% accuracy with LSTMs and 93.79% with Bi-LSTMs. Ali et al. (2022) observe 88.04% accuracy for LSTMs and 94.84% for Bi-LSTMs.

Decision trees and Random Forest are popular machine learning methods for classification and regression. Decision trees split data through binary decisions. Each node selects a feature, and each branch reflects the outcome. Although easy to interpret, deep or complex trees often overfit (Baygin et al., 2021; Mohi ud Din and Jayanthy, 2023). Random Forest aggregates multiple decision trees. It trains each tree on random data subsets and random features. This approach reduces correlation among trees, lowers overfitting, and boosts performance. In the reviewed studies, decision trees achieved 82.40% accuracy in Baygin et al. (2021) and 80% in Mohi-ud Din et al. (2023). Random Forest performed at 43.03% in Tasnim et al. (2022), 90.59% in Tawhid et al. (2021), 98.06% in Jayawardana et al. (2019), and 99.75% in de Oliveira Silva et al. (2024) with a configuration of 500 trees.

K-Nearest Neighbors (KNN) demonstrates high effectiveness in practice, despite its structural simplicity. It is an instance-based classifier that does not assume a specific data distribution shape. KNN stores training data and classifies a new instance by checking the classes of its closest neighbors. The parameter k defines how many neighbors the algorithm considers. KNN performs well in EEG-based ASD diagnosis. Rechal et al. (2021) reported 94.58% accuracy, Tawhid et al. (2021) reached 92.29%, and Mohi ud Din and Jayanthy (2023) obtained 93%. These results confirm KNN's robustness in complex tasks.

Logistic Regression is a common choice for binary classification due to its simplicity and effectiveness. It can also extend to multiple classes. Despite its basic structure, it delivers robust and interpretable models. In EEG signal analysis for ASD, Logistic Regression performs well. Baygin et al. (2021) achieved 87.50% accuracy, Tawhid et al. (2021) reached 94.95%, and Mohi ud Din and Jayanthy (2023) reported 93%. These findings show its competitiveness compared to advanced methods and highlight its relevance when researchers value interpretability and simplicity. They also confirm its usefulness for ASD diagnosis from EEG data (Jayawardana et al., 2019).

Support Vector Machine (SVM) is a high-performance classifier that constructs accurate decision boundaries. Its core principle involves finding the optimal hyperplane that maximizes the margin between classes, improving generalization and robustness. SVM handles both linear and nonlinear classification through kernel functions. For example, the radial basis function (RBF) maps data to a higher-dimensional space, enabling linear separation there. The polynomial kernel captures complex interactions among variables with polynomial transformations. In EEG-based ASD diagnosis, SVM often produces accuracy above 90% (Oh et al., 2021; Peng et al., 2021; Rechal et al., 2021; Wadhera et al., 2023). However, results vary. Tasnim et al. (2022) only reported 56.62% accuracy. This contrast highlights the importance of choosing an appropriate kernel and tuning the model to each dataset and context.

Dimensionality reduction techniques and statistical methods, such as Linear Discriminant Analysis (LDA), play a key role in boosting machine learning model efficiency and accuracy. They are especially relevant with high-dimensional data. LDA identifies a linear combination of features that maximizes class separation and provides optimal discrimination. This approach often highlights features that distinguish specific brain activity patterns, improving diagnostic accuracy and reliability. Recent studies show variable results with LDA, revealing the impact of data characteristics and experimental choices. Tawhid et al. (2021) reported 89.97% accuracy, Tasnim et al. (2022) reached 66.36%, and Melinda et al. (2023) attained 99%. These differences confirm the influence of model configuration, data quality, and context. Researchers must adjust LDA carefully when analyzing complex signals, such as EEG data for ASD diagnosis.

The Naïve Bayes (NB) classifier relies on Bayes' theorem. It is known for its simplicity and effectiveness in classification. The model calculates class probabilities based on input features while assuming conditional independence. Although this assumption does not always hold in real scenarios, it simplifies calculations and lowers computational costs. Despite that limitation, NB often delivers competitive results. Tawhid et al. (2021) demonstrated its utility in EEG signal analysis with 72.09% accuracy. This performance, combined with high speed and the capacity to handle large datasets, makes NB a strong candidate for neurophysiological signal classification.

The use of classifiers for EEG-based early ASD diagnosis shows a promising bridge between technology and neuroscience. These algorithms convert raw data into meaningful information, revealing subtle patterns in brain signals. They add fresh perspectives to our understanding and detection of ASD. Machine learning and AI offer various levels of sophistication. Each approach balances accuracy, efficiency, and clinical utility. Researchers should choose the most appropriate classifier based on data characteristics and study goals. Combining complementary methods and advanced techniques can boost model performance. This collaboration leads to more precise diagnoses and deeper insights into ASD. Ongoing progress in classification methods, aligned with data specifics, is essential to strengthen diagnostic capability and advance computational neuroscience.

3. Limitations

Despite encouraging findings, several limitations may influence how we interpret and apply these results. EEG-based ASD detection studies highlight recurring challenges that can reduce model effectiveness and generalizability. One concern is reliance on multimodal data, like EEG with eye tracking, which demands both modalities simultaneously. Many clinical settings lack the needed infrastructure.

Computational complexity also matters. Complex methods, such as convolutional neural networks, need significant computational power. This requirement may hinder real-world deployment in clinics that value speed and efficiency. Additional hardware optimization, such as using GPUs (graphic processing units), and the inherent complexity of these models can complicate real-time implementation. This issue affects immediate clinical utility and integration with continuous monitoring systems.

Another major constraint involves band and channel choices. Many models rely on specific frequency bands and particular channels. This dependence limits their use in other configurations or populations. It also reduces model generalization and complicates adaptation to varied clinical scenarios. Individual differences in EEG signals further affect model accuracy. Some studies report that sensitivity changes with different levels of ASD severity, indicating a need to tailor models to distinct patient profiles.

Result generalization remains a key concern. Researchers often test methods on unique datasets that do not capture the range of variation in broader populations or clinical environments. This narrow focus restricts a model's applicability. In addition, differences in how specialists define and interpret EEG abnormalities cause inconsistencies in data analysis. This challenge complicates result comparisons across studies and weakens their reliability.

Feature selection and interpretation also pose problems. Researchers may not capture all relevant EEG variables. They may include redundant features that lower model performance. Many studies have too few participants to reflect the diversity in EEG patterns and reactions to stimuli. This shortcoming limits external validity and reduces overall generalizability.

In summary, EEG-based ASD detection research encounters hurdles such as limited data availability and diversity, high computational demands, dependence on specific bands or channels, and individual EEG variation. Generalizing findings across diverse contexts stands as another major obstacle. Researchers must overcome these issues to strengthen the reliability and usefulness of ASD detection models in clinical practice. This progress would support a more robust and universal approach.

4. Conclusion

We apply EEG signals with machine learning for the early diagnosis of ASD. This approach holds transformative potential for clinical practice. It promises quicker and more precise diagnoses. The methods described show the ability of computational models to detect subtle patterns in EEG signals and identify features that may point to ASD. We also integrate other technologies, such as eye tracking and audio and video signals. This multimodal strategy expands these models, enriches analyses, and raises diagnostic accuracy.

Preprocessing stands out as a key factor for successful early ASD diagnostics. We use bandpass filters, windowing, and the Fourier Transform to focus on important frequencies and remove noise. Independent Component Analysis and the Short-Time Fourier Transform help isolate the temporal and frequency aspects of signals. Wavelet transforms target both temporal and frequency data, leading to a more detailed view of EEG fluctuations. These steps extract essential features and allow computational models to detect and distinguish ASD-specific patterns.

Despite this potential, we face several challenges in clinical practice. High computational demands, along with the need for certain data types and specific band or channel setups, limit broader adoption. Individual EEG variations further reduce accuracy. A lack of standardized criteria for anomaly detection and the use of small, unrepresentative databases also hinder progress. We must solve these issues to ensure effective and adaptable models across diverse clinical settings.

Future research must address these gaps. We need more robust and diverse databases. We must optimize models for real-time performance across different clinical environments. We also need to adapt these models for distinct patient profiles to boost diagnostic accuracy, especially given the variations seen in ASD.

Therefore, advanced classification methods, complementary approaches, and improved EEG signal preprocessing techniques hold a vital role in optimizing ASD diagnosis. They also drive progress in computational neuroscience. Overcoming these barriers leads to more effective and accessible solutions. These solutions benefit individuals with ASD and their families and expand scientific knowledge of the disorder.

Acknowledgment(s)

This study was partially financed by the Financiadora de Estudos e Projetos – Brasil (Finep). We are also grateful to Coordenação de Aperfeiçoamento de Pessoal de Nível Superior – Brazil (CAPES), Fundação de Amparo à Ciência e Tecnologia do Estado de Pernambuco – Brazil (FACEPE), and the National Council for Scientific and Technological Development – Brazil (CNPq) for the partial financial support.

Disclosure Statement

No authors have financial or non-financial conflicts of interest to declare.

References

Abdulhay, E., Alafeef, M., Hadoush, H., Venkataraman, V. and Arunkumar, N. (2022). EMD-based analysis of complexity with dissociated EEG amplitude and frequency information: A data-driven robust tool for autism diagnosis compared to multi-scale entropy approach. *Mathematical Biosciences and Engineering*, *19*(5), 5031–5054.

Ali, N.A., Syafeeza, A., Jaafar, A. and Nor, N.K. (2022). ConvNet BiLSTM for ASD classification on EEG brain signals. *International Journal of Online and Biomedical Engineering*, *18*(11).

Bairagi, V.K. and Elgandelwar, S.M. (2023). Early diagnosis of Alzheimer disease using EEG signals: The role of pre-processing. *International Journal of Biomedical Engineering and Technology*, *41*(4), 317–339.

Baygin, M., Dogan, S., Tuncer, T., Datta Barua, P., Faust, O., Arunkumar, N., Abdulhay, E.W., Palmer, E.E. and Acharya, U.R. 2021. Automated ASD detection using hybrid deep lightweight features extracted from EEG signals. *Computers in Biology and Medicine*, *134*, 104548. https://www.sciencedirect.com/science/article/pii/S0010482521003425

Chen, H., Gaoxiang, O. and Li, X. (2023). Extracting temporal-spectral-spatial representation of EEG using self-supervised learning for the identification of children with ASD. In: *2023 IEEE 13th International Conference on CYBER Technology in Automation, Control, and Intelligent Systems* (*CYBER*), pp. 1263–1266. IEEE.

de Oliveira Silva, A.S., Fonseca, F.S., Muniz, M.V.S., de Melo, A.M.N., Machado, W.G., de Santana, M.A. and Carneiro, J. (2024). Enhancing ASD diagnosis with low-density EEG and machine learning. In: *XXIX Conference Congresso Brasileiro de Engenharia Biomédica* (*CBEB* 2024) at Ribeirão Preto. ResearchGate.

Han, J., Jiang, G., Ouyang, G. and Li, X. (2022). A multimodal approach for identifying autism spectrum disorders in children. *IEEE Transactions on Neural Systems and Rehabilitation Engineering*, *30*, 2003–2011.

Ieracitano, C., Mammone, N., Bramanti, A., Hussain, A. and Morabito, F.C. (2019). A convolutional neural network approach for classification of dementia stages based on 2D-spectral representation of EEG recordings. *Neurocomputing*, *323*, 96–107.

Jayawardana, Y., Jaime, M., Thapaliya, S. and Jayarathna, S. (2019). Electroencephalogram (EEG) for delineating objective measure of autism spectrum disorder (ASD) (extended version). *arXiv preprint arXiv:1907.01515*.

Kansara, N., Rajkumar, A., Dharmale, P. and Khadtare, M. (2024). Enhancing autism spectrum disorder recognition in EEG data through filtering-driven CNN approach. In: *2024 IEEE International Conference on Consumer Electronics* (*ICCE*), pp. 1–7. IEEE.

Maestro, S., Muratori, F., Cesari, A., Cavallaro, M., Paziente, A., Pecini, C., Grassi, C., Manfredi, A. and Sommario, C. (2005). Course of autism signs in the first year of life. *Psychopathology*, *38*, 26–31.

Melinda, M., Maulisa, O., Nabila, N.H., Yunidar, Y. and Enriko, I.K.A. (2023). Classification of EEG signal using independent component analysis and discrete wavelet transform based on linear discriminant analysis. *JOIV: International Journal on Informatics Visualization*, *7*(3), 830–838.

Menaka, R., Karthik, R., Saranya, S., Niranjan, M. and Kabilan, S. (2024). An improved AlexNet model and cepstral coefficient-based classification of autism using EEG. *Clinical EEG and Neuroscience*, *55*(1), 43–51.

Mohi-ud Din, Q. and Jayanthy, A. (2021). Detection of autism spectrum disorder from EEG signals using pre-trained deep convolution neural networks. In: *2021 Seventh International Conference on Bio Signals, Images, and Instrumentation* (*ICBSII*), pp. 1–5. IEEE.

Mohi-ud Din, Q. and Jayanthy, A. (2023). Detection of autism spectrum disorder by feature extraction of EEG signals and machine learning classifiers. *Biomedical Engineering: Applications, Basis, and Communications*, *35*(1), 2250046.

Napolitano, A., Schiavi, S., Rosa, P.L., Rossi-Espagnet, M.C., Petrillo, S., Bottino, F., Tagliente, E., Longo, D., Lupi, E., Casula, L., Valeri, G., Piemonte, F., Trezza, V. and Vicari, S. (2022). Sex differences in autism spectrum disorder: Diagnostic, neurobiological, and behavioral features. *Frontiers in Psychiatry*, *13*.

Oh, S.L., Jahmunah, V., Arunkumar, N., Abdulhay, E.W., Gururajan, R., Adib, N., Ciaccio, E.J., Cheong, K.H. and Acharya, U.R. (2021). A novel automated autism spectrum disorder detection system. *Complex and Intelligent Systems*, *7*(5), 2399–2413.

Peng, S., Xu, R., Yi, X., Hu, X., Liu, L. and Liu, L. (2021). Early screening of children with autism spectrum disorder based on electroencephalogram signal feature selection with L1-norm regularization. *Frontiers in Human Neuroscience*, *15*, 656578.

Peter-Derex, L., Berthomier, C., Taillard, J., Berthomier, P., Bouet, R., Mattout, J., Brandewinder, M. and Bastuji, H. (2021). Automatic analysis of single-channel sleep EEG in a large spectrum of sleep disorders. *Journal of Clinical Sleep Medicine*, *17*(3), 393–402.

Radhakrishnan, M., Ramamurthy, K., Kothandaraman, A., Madaan, G. and Machavaram, H. (2021). Investigating EEG signals of autistic individuals using detrended fluctuation analysis. *Traitement du Signal*, *38*(5).

Radhakrishnan, M., Boruah, S. and Ramamurthy, K. (2022). EEG-based anomaly detection for autistic kids: A pilot study. *Traitement du Signal*, *39*(3).

Rechal, T.R., Kumar, P.R. and Khaleelulla, S.E. (2021). A feasibility approach in diagnosing ASD with P300 via machine learning classification approach using BCI. In: *2021 International Conference on Computing, Communication, and Intelligent Systems* (*ICCCIS*), pp. 557–562. IEEE.

Sanabria-Barradas, B., Sanei, S. and Granados-Ramos, D.E. (2022). A hybrid tensor factorization–singular spectrum analysis approach for ERP-based assessment of autism in children. In: *2022 30th European Signal Processing Conference* (*EUSIPCO*), pp. 1193–1197. IEEE.

Tasnim, N., Halder, J., Ahmed, S. and Fattah, S.A. (2022). An approach for analyzing cognitive behavior of autism spectrum disorder using P300 BCI data. In: *2022 IEEE Region 10 Symposium* (*TENSYMP*), pp. 1–6. IEEE.

Tatum, W.O., Rubboli, G., Kaplan, P.W., Mirsatari, S., Radhakrishnan, K., Gloss, D., Caboclo, L., Drislane, F., Koutroumanidis, M., Schomer, D., et al. (2018). Clinical utility of EEG in diagnosing and monitoring epilepsy in adults. *Clinical Neurophysiology*, *129*(5), 1056–1082.

Tawhid, M.N.A., Siuly, S., Wang, H., Whittaker, F., Wang, K. and Zhang, Y. (2021). A spectrogram image-based intelligent technique for automatic detection of autism spectrum disorder from EEG. *PLOS ONE*, *16*(6), e0253094.

Tong, W., Yue, W., Chen, F., Shi, W., Zhang, L. and Wan, J. (2024). MSE-VGG: A novel deep learning approach based on EEG for rapid ischemic stroke detection. *Sensors*, *24*(13), 4234.

Wadhera, T., Bedi, J. and Sharma, S. (2023). Autism spectrum disorder prediction using bidirectional stacked gated recurrent unit with time-distributor wrapper: An EEG study. *Neural Computing and Applications*, *35*(13), 9803–9818.

6 Enhancing EEG-Based ASD Detection Using Wavelet Transforms and Hybrid Deep Learning Models

Maíra Araújo de Santana[1], Jordana Leandro Seixas[2], Flávio Secco Fonseca[2], Arthur Moreira Nogueira de Melo[1], Camila Xavier de Medeiros[1], Wesley Gregório Machado[1] and Wellington Pinheiro dos Santos[1,2]

This chapter investigates the use of an integrated approach combining wavelet transform and a hybrid architecture to improve the accuracy and reliability of Autism Spectrum Disorder (ASD) diagnosis using electroencephalography (EEG) data. Wavelet transforms are employed to convert the EEG signals to images, which are then processed by an architecture with a pre-trained convolutional neural network for feature extraction and a classic classifier to capture intricate patterns of brain activity. The overall performance indicates room for improvement since the best classification accuracy was 69.047% by using LeNet combined with Random Forest. Part of this performance is justified by the quality of the database, which has missing data and little variability. However, this study already demonstrates good potential for an AI-supported approach in reducing false negative rates during the diagnostic process.

1. Introduction

Autism Spectrum Disorder (ASD) is a group of neurodevelopmental-related conditions that affect about 1 in 100 children worldwide (WHO, 2023). Characteristics of ASD may include but are not limited to hyperfocus, difficulties with social interaction, communication, and repetitive behaviors (WHO, 2023). These factors are usually present since early childhood, but are difficult to differentiate, leading to late diagnosis of autism (Hus and Segal, 2021). However, accurate and early diagnosis of ASD is critical for ensuring timely intervention and support, which can significantly enhance developmental outcomes for individuals (WHO, 2023; Hus and Segal, 2021).

[1] Universidade Federal de Pernambuco, Brazil.
[2] Universidade de Pernambuco, Brazil.
* Corresponding author: maira.araujosantana@ufpe.br.

DOI: 10.1201/9781003531418-6

Electroencephalography (EEG) has emerged as a non-invasive, cost-effective, and widely accessible tool for studying brain activity, including neurodiverse brains. Yet, the complexity of EEG signals presents significant challenges in extracting meaningful patterns that can assist in clinical decision-making (Bouazizi and Ltifi, 2024; Chaddad et al., 2023). In recent years, artificial intelligence (AI) has revolutionized several domains of healthcare, offering advanced analytical capabilities to interpret complex datasets (Chaddad et al., 2023; Andrade et al., 2020; Oliveira et al., 2020; Santana et al., 2020a,b; Santana et al., 2018; Cruz et al., 2018; Barbosa et al., 2020, 2021; Gomes et al., 2020).

For ASD diagnosis, AI-driven approaches have shown promise in identifying subtle, clinically relevant patterns in EEG signals. Among these, deep neural networks (DNNs) have demonstrated exceptional performance in learning hierarchical representations of data, while wavelet transforms have proven effective in capturing both time and frequency-domain features of EEG signals (Chaddad et al., 2023; Santana et al., 2023).

This chapter explores an integrated approach combining wavelet transform and DNNs to enhance the accuracy and reliability of ASD diagnosis using EEG data. The wavelet transform is utilized to convert EEG signals into multi-resolution images that are used as input of a pre-trained DNN to build a robust feature set that aims to encapsulate the intricate dynamics of brain activity.

By leveraging the strengths of wavelet analysis and deep learning, this approach aims to address the limitations of traditional processing methods. This chapter will review some relevant literature findings, provide an overview of the methodology, highlight key findings, and discuss the implications of this approach for advancing ASD diagnostics and broader applications in neurodevelopmental research.

2. Literature Related to AI Applied to ASD

In recent years, several studies have investigated the use of machine learning techniques and DNNs for the detection of ASD, especially with neuroimaging data. Kashef (2022) proposed an improved convolutional neural network (ECNN) model to identify functional connectivity patterns in the brain of individuals with ASD using fMRI (Functional Magnetic Resonance Imaging) data. The model demonstrated an accuracy of 80% and superior computational efficiency to previous approaches, such as those based on Support Vector Machines (SVM) and Gaussian Naïve Bayes (GNB), applied to large databases such as ABIDE (Kashef, 2022). Complementarily, Deng et al. (2022) used a 3D-CNN model to diagnose ASD with fMRI, achieving 74.53% accuracy when combining different brain regions, indicating that combining multiple brain regions improves accuracy compared to using these regions alone (Deng et al., 2022).

In addition to the use of neuroimaging, other works have focused on the analysis of biometric signals and speech data to diagnose ASD. Sai et al. (2024) explored the use of raw speech data from children for the automatic detection of ASD, employing the fast Fourier transform (STFT) with custom CNNs, achieving up to 99.1% accuracy when using data augmentation techniques (Sai et al., 2024). In turn, Cetintas et al. (2023) proposed a hybrid CNN model based on pupil diameter variation to detect ASD and classify the severity of the condition. Using multimodal feature fusion methods, the study obtained an accuracy of 95.33%, reinforcing the viability of visual biometric parameters as efficient diagnostic markers for ASD (Cetintas et al., 2023).

The study by Peketi and Dhok (2023) investigated the complexity of detecting the P300 signal in individuals with ASD, highlighting its importance for brain-computer interfaces (BCIs). However, its detection is challenging due to the low amplitude and high latency, common in signals of people with ASD. To overcome these difficulties, the researchers proposed the use of Variational Mode Decomposition (VMD), an advanced technique for dealing with non-stationary signals. This innovative approach achieved accuracy of 91.12% in EEG analysis, which was considered better than other state-of-the-art approaches (Peketi and Dhok, 2023). This study connects with the work of Kang (2020), who also used EEG to detect ASD, but incorporating eye-tracking. By combining EEG and eye-tracking, the researchers reached accuracies up to 85.44%, and they identified specific brain and behavioral patterns, suggesting that the fusion of these signals can increase knowledge about ASD diagnosis (Kang, 2020).

Abdulhay et al. (2023) also presented an innovative approach by exploring the EEG ripple range (75–250 Hz) to diagnose ASD. Using power spectra and Shannon entropy, the study achieved an impressive accuracy of 98.9%, highlighting the effectiveness of this underexplored range in distinguishing between individuals with ASD and neurotypicals (Abdulhay et al., 2023). This proposal complements the work of Kang (2020), which also focuses on improving ASD diagnosis from EEG, but with an emphasis on combining multiple data sources, such as eye tracking, to increase diagnostic accuracy. In the same context, Din and Jayanthy (2022) applied the Second-Order Wavelet Transform (WST) along with DNNs for the analysis of EEG signals. Using techniques such as Long Short Term Memory (LSTM) and CNNs, the authors achieved accuracies of 94% and 92%, respectively, highlighting the potential of WST coefficients as effective biomarkers for ASD, further extending previous approaches and allowing a more detailed analysis of brain activity (Din and Jayanthy, 2022).

Finally, Al-Qazzaz et al. (2024) proposed a hybrid model using pre-trained CNNs, achieving an accuracy of 87.8% when combined with SVM. This study reinforces the growing trend of applying hybrid methods based on convolutional neural networks for the analysis of EEG signals in the diagnosis of ASD. The combination of CNNs with SVM showed promise in improving diagnostic accuracy, especially when considering the heterogeneity of ASD and the need for more effective and accessible diagnostic methods (Al-Qazzaz et al., 2024).

These studies, taken together, reflect the evolution of machine learning techniques applied to the diagnosis of ASD. The use of advanced approaches, such as adaptive signal decomposition, EEG ripple analysis and the implementation of DNNs, have shown great potential to increase the accuracy and sensitivity of the diagnosis. In addition, the fusion of different data sources, such as EEG and eye tracking, demonstrates the increasing sophistication of diagnostic tools, which seek to identify ASD earlier and more efficiently, promoting a significant advance in the field of non-invasive and automated detection of the disorder.

3. An Approach to EEG Analysis of ASD Subjects

The study presented in this chapter consists of an evaluation of the performance of a method proposed by Santana (2023) for signal analysis, including EEG signals (Santana, 2023; Santana and Santos, 2024;, Santana et al., 2023). In this approach, raw signals are converted into images by wavelet transform. These images are then used as input to a hybrid architecture composed of a CNN to extract features and a classical classification algorithm. In this study, different common classifiers in literature were investigated to assess which would be most suitable for differentiating data from people with and without ASD. The proposed methodology is illustrated in Figure 1.

3.1 Database

To perform the experiments, we used Dataset 1 from the Sheffield database (Dickinson, 2022), in which the researchers used a Biosemi Active Two EEG system to obtain EEG signals from 56 subjects, aged 18 to 68; 28 with ASD and 28 without ASD. They collected EEG data for 150 seconds, with eyes closed, at rest, and during visual stimulation. The reference channel was Cz, and the signals were filtered with a band-pass filter of 0.01 and 140 Hz. Most participants had data from a 64-electrode setup (Dickinson, 2022), while some had data from 128 electrodes (Oostenveld and Praamstra, 2001). Therefore, the 128-electrode assemblies were readjusted to 64-electrode

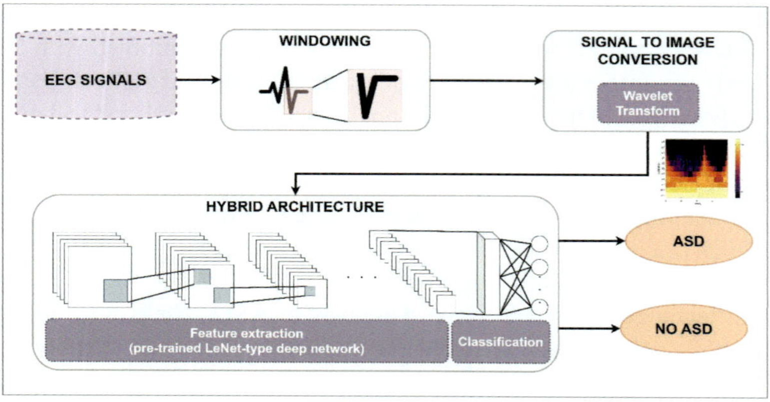

Fig. 1 Proposed method to process EEG data to differentiate subjects into ASD and no ASD groups.

assemblies before analysis to obtain a better comparison between the groups. EEGLAB (Delorme and Makeig, 2004) was used to filter the continuous data with band margins and transition passband of 1 Hz each. Data corrupted by anomalies were excluded and the data were subsequently made available with the sampling frequency reduced to 512 Hz.

During the analysis of the database, we identified some issues that are important to highlight. The first is the presence of missing electrodes (Figure 2). This is common in EEG databases due to technical problems and possible participant movements. However, these missing electrodes create gaps in the data, resulting in an incomplete view of brain activity. The second problem is the lack of standardization in the positioning of the electrodes, as it can affect the accuracy of measurements and interpretation of brain activity. Another difficulty is the use of high-density electrode systems. Although they offer wider coverage and better resolution, they also make the data more complex, generating a large volume of information that can overload computers, making it difficult to analyze brain patterns.

The organization of the database for processing began with the conversion of the files from the original acquisition formats (.set and .fdt) to .edf because it can handle many channels of temporal data (Kemp and Olivan, 2003). Then, we converted the files with the EEG signal data to .csv using Python script 3.11.1 (Van Rossum and Drake, 2009). This step made the signals easier to process in different software.

The first step of processing was handling the missing data previously reported. To fill in the dataset we applied an interpolation method called Inverse Distance Weighting (IDW). However, in this version of the formula,

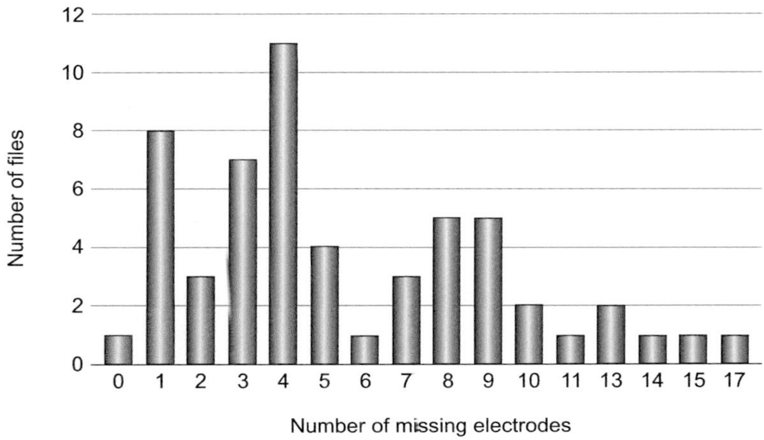

Fig. 2 Distribution of EEG files according to the quantity of missing data points. Each bar corresponds to the amount of absent data.

the inverse of the distance was replaced by the negative exponential to reduce computational cost and avoid division by zero. Its exploratory goal is to reduce error propagation by performing a single interpolation. To obtain the respective coordinates (x, y), we used the GIMP software (version 2.10.34) (Oliver et al., 2006). With this, we calculated the distance between each point using Equation 1, which applies the Pythagorean theorem (Maor, 2019) to find the distance between any two points (d_{ab}), where a and b are the points, x_a and y_a are the coordinates of point a, and x_b and y_b are the coordinates of point b.

$$d_{ab} = \sqrt{\{(x_b - x_a)^2 + (y_b - y_a)^2\}} \quad ...(1)$$

After finding this distance, we used Equation 2 to fill in the missing channel (p_j), where p_i is the data of a non-missing channel and m is the amount of considered neighbors.

$$p_j = \frac{\sum_{i=1}^{m} (p_i^e)^{-d_{ij}}}{\sum_{i=1}^{m} e^{-d_{ij}}} \quad ...(2)$$

With the completed dataset, we conducted a windowing process, splitting the signals using a 5s window with 1s overlap. Then, we converted each piece of signal into image using Fast Wavelet Transform (FWT), applying the Mallat algorithm with 10 filter banks of the Daubechies 8 (db8) family (Mallat, 1989). We generated the images from the plot of the coefficients resulting from the FWT. The signal channels were concatenated before applying the transform, so that 1 image was built for each signal window, all saved in .jpeg format. This step was implemented in Octave, version 5.1.0 (Eaton, 2019), and examples of the images can be seen in Figure 3. At the end of this process, the dataset had 503 images, 251 with ASD and 252 of control group.

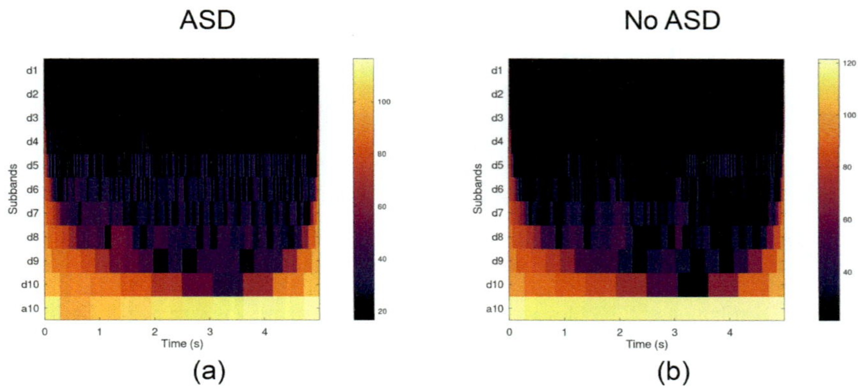

Fig. 3 Examples of images generated by the Wavelet Transform applied to EEG signals.

3.2 Hybrid Architecture

Adopting a hybrid architecture based on deep transfer learning and shallow classifiers allows reducing the computational complexity associated with training large image databases, as it minimizes the problem of adjusting the various training parameters, in addition to combining well-established state-of-the-art learning models.

Thus, we performed the feature extraction of the images using a pre-trained CNN. In this study, we used a LeNet with 7 layers (2 convolutional, 2 pooling, and 3 fully connected), average pooling and ReLu activation function (LeCun et al., 1998; Lang et al., 2019). According to the principle of transfer learning, the deep network model was trained with the MNIST database (Deng, 2012), which is robust, multiclass and well classified by the LeNet network. In this configuration, the network extracts 500 features from each input image.

To perform the training and evaluation of the tested configurations, the dataset was initially divided into a part for training-validation and another for testing. We used 75% of the original set for training and 25% for testing. The training-validation set is used to evaluate the classification performance of all experimented classifier settings. We assessed classification performance by conducting each training using the *k*-fold cross-validation method with $k = 10$ and 30 runs of each classifier configuration. Thus, the training results presented here consist of the average of the performances obtained in these repetitions.

To build the classification layer of the proposed hybrid architecture, with a pre-trained deep network for feature extraction and a classical method for classification (Figure 1), we assessed the performances of the following classifiers: Random Forest (10, 20, 50, 100, 150, 200, 250, and 300 trees), SVM (kernels: linear, polynomial of degree 2, and RBF with gamma 0.01, 0.25, and 0.50), J48 decision tree, and Bayesian networks (Bayes Network and Naive Bayes). We conducted the experiments with several architectures using their respective Java implementations in Weka software, version 3.8 (Witten and Frank, 2005).

We compared the classification performances in terms of accuracy, kappa statistics, sensitivity, specificity and area under the ROC curve (AUC-ROC) to define the most appropriate model for differentiating signals from people with and without ASD. With the best model defined, we used this algorithm to classify the data from the previously separated test set. This step is important to evaluate the ability of this model to generalize the knowledge about the data, that is, its performance when submitted to new data.

3.3 Results and Discussion

In this section, we will present the computational results obtained during the training and testing stages.

3.3.1 Training and Validation

Table 1 presents the performance of the evaluated LeNet-based architectures. The quality of the binary classification of patients with and without ASD in the EEG signals was measured from the arithmetic means and standard deviations of the five metrics: accuracy, kappa, sensitivity, specificity, and AUC-ROC. The table highlights the classifier with the best overall performance, whose choice considers the mean and standard deviation values of each metric.

From these results, we noticed that the adopted approach did not favor the classification of ASD from this data. Despite the unsatisfactory performance, the sensitivity reached expressive values. Considering the results in Table 1, in this dataset represented by LeNet, the best classification performance was achieved by the J48 classifier with an average accuracy of 60.96%, kappa index of 0.2198, sensitivity of 0.7208, specificity of 0.4992, and average AUC-ROC of 0.6391. The other classifiers: Random Forest (10 trees), SVM (RBF 0.25 and RBF 0.50), and Bayes Network also had similar performances to J48.

Table 1 Performance of different LeNet-based architectures for binary classification with and without ASD from EEG.

Classifiers		*Accuracy (%)*	*Kappa Index*	*Sensitivity*	*Specificity*	*ROC Area*
Random Forest	10	59.4595 ± 7.3885	0.1933 ± 0.1473	0.7368 ± 0.1053	0.4327 ± 0.1072	0.6260 ± 0.0878
	20	57.8947 ± 7.3991	0.1579 ± 0.1474	0.7368 ± 0.1037	0.4211 ± 0.1140	0.6260 ± 0.0871
	50	57.8947 ± 7.1503	0.1579 ± 0.1420	0.7368 ± 0.1006	0.4211 ± 0.1159	0.6191 ± 0.0901
	100	57.8947 ± 6.9870	0.1579 ± 0.1388	0.7368 ± 0.1010	0.4211 ± 0.1076	0.6163 ± 0.0873
	150	57.8954 ± 7.0669	0.1590 ± 0.1402	0.7554 ± 0.0986	0.4036 ± 0.1092	0.6065 ± 0.0879
	200	57.5538 ± 7.3056	0.1521 ± 0.1451	0.7565 ± 0.1033	0.3956 ± 0.1107	0.6042 ± 0.0877
	250	57.6283 ± 7.2423	0.1536 ± 0.1437	0.7593 ± 0.1013	0.3943 ± 0.1100	0.6042 ± 0.0886
	300	57.6050 ± 7.2806	0.1531 ± 0.1445	0.7622 ± 0.0990	0.3910 ± 0.1101	0.6041 ± 0.0889
SVM	Linear	53.7181 ± 7.2925	0.0749 ± 0.1457	0.6257 ± 0.1221	0.4492 ± 0.1102	0.5375 ± 0.0729
	Poli 2	56.2183 ± 7.5033	0.1244 ± 0.1502	0.5350 ± 0.1235	0.5894 ± 0.1056	0.5622 ± 0.0751
	RBF 0.01	56.7639 ± 6.9106	0.1358 ± 0.1380	0.6156 ± 0.1181	0.5203 ± 0.1162	0.5680 ± 0.0691
	RBF 0.25	59.3976 ± 6.7940	0.1891 ± 0.1344	0.8458 ± 0.0908	0.3433 ± 0.1068	0.5946 ± 0.0671
	RBF 0.5	60.7361 ± 6.5286	0.2160 ± 0.1294	0.8754 ± 0.0875	0.3408 ± 0.1076	0.6081 ± 0.0647
J48	-	**60.9659 ± 7.1417**	**0.2198 ± 0.1425**	**0.7208 ± 0.1938**	**0.4992 ± 0.1719**	**0.6391 ± 0.0783**
Bayes Network	-	59.9697 ± 7.0253	0.2005 ± 0.1394	0.8300 ± 0.0908	0.3707 ± 0.1028	0.6384 ± 0.872
Naive Bayes	-	1.0244 ± 1.6162	0.8571 ± 0.3564	0.9674 ± 0.1194	0.0000 ± 0.0000	0.5024 ± 0.0105

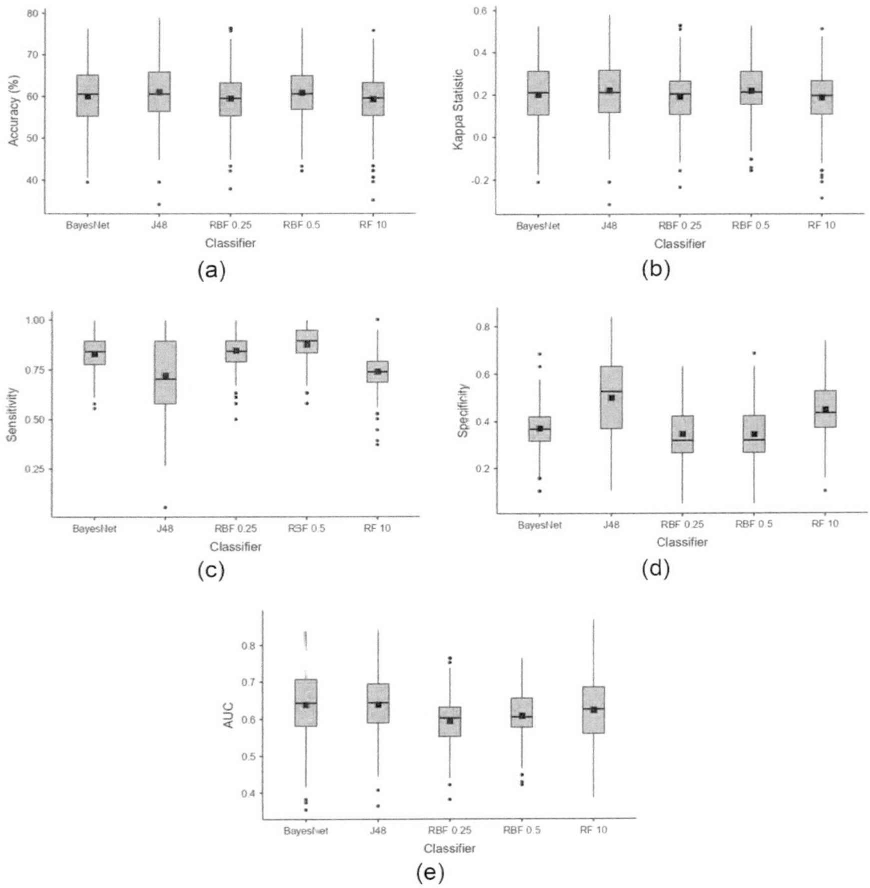

Fig. 4 Performance of the best configurations in classifying patients with and without ASD from EEG. The statistical behavior of each classifier is presented in terms of: (a) accuracy, (b) Kappa, (c) sensitivity, (d) specificity, and (e) AUC-ROC.

To better compare the classifiers, observing the statistical behavior of their performances, we used the boxplot graphs presented in Figure 4. A graph was plotted for each metric with the results obtained from the 30 executions of the training with cross-validation. It is worth noting that we plotted only the results of the top 5 classifiers: J48, Random Forest (10 trees), SVM (RBF 0.25 and RBF 0.50) and Bayes Network. From these graphs we can see that for all metrics the performances of the classifiers were statistically equivalent. For this reason, all 5 models were evaluated in the testing stage.

3.3.2 Testing

The testing phase was run for each model only once with 25% of the data, separated from the original base, without contact with the training stage. Table 2 shows the performance of the best configurations found during training. It is possible to observe that the performances were similar to those obtained in training, with equivalent values between the classifiers.

Table 2 Performance of the top 5 LeNet-based architectures on testing with new data.

Metrics	*RF 10 trees*	*SVM RBF 0.25*	*SVM RBF 0.5*	*J48*	*Bayes Network*
Accuracy	**69.947%**	66.667%	67.460%	59.525%	68.254%
Kappa Index	**0.381**	0.333	0.349	0.190	0.365
Sensitivity	**0.690**	0.667	0.675	0.595	0.683
Specificity	**0.690**	0.667	0.675	0.595	0.683
ROC Area	**0.696**	0.667	0.675	0.654	0.696

Random Forest (RF) achieved an accuracy of 69.047%, a difference of 0.793% compared to the second best, Bayes Network. Despite superior results, both RF and Bayes Network and the other models tested presented a low Kappa index, below 0.4, indicating low agreement in the results. The other metrics of the tested classifiers varied between 0.595 and 0.696, indicating an intermediate performance. SVM RBF, with gamma of 0.5, presented an accuracy of 66.66%, a satisfactory performance compared to the two best results. SVM RBF with gamma of 0.25 demonstrated a slightly lower accuracy compared to the configuration with gamma 0.5, which was expected due to the smaller number of parameters.

Unlike the training, J48 classifier presented the worst performance among the five models, with a kappa of 0.1, accuracy of 59.52%, ROC area of 0.65, sensitivity and specificity of 0.59. However, these values are within the range estimated in training (average ± standard deviation).

Table 3 presents the confusion matrices of these top 5 classifiers, detailing how each model correctly or incorrectly classified ASD and non-ASD instances. Analyzing the results we may see that, with the exception of classifier J48, which had difficulty correctly identifying ASD instances, the other models showed good performance in classifying data belonging to the ASD category.

Table 3 Confusion Matrices of the best results.

Classifiers	*Category*	*ASD*	*No ASD*
Random Forest 10 trees	ASD	50	13
	No ASD	26	37
SVM RBF 0.25	ASD	58	5
	No ASD	37	26
SVM RBF 0.5	ASD	59	4
	No ASD	37	26
J48	ASD	32	30
	No ASD	20	43
Bayes Network	ASD	57	6
	No ASD	34	29

The greatest variation between classifiers occurred in the non-ASD category. RF, which performed best overall, correctly classified 37 of the 63 non-ASD instances. In comparison, SVM RBF models with different gamma settings performed worse in this category, correctly classifying only 26 of the 63 instances.

4. Final Considerations

This chapter explored the integration of wavelet transform and deep neural networks as a promising approach to enhance the accuracy of ASD diagnosis using EEG data. By leveraging the multi-resolution capabilities of wavelet analysis and the hierarchical representation learning of DNNs, this methodology aimed to address critical challenges associated with the complexity of EEG signals in neurodevelopmental research.

Despite its potential, the results of this study reveal areas for further improvement. While the RF classifier achieved the highest accuracy (69.047%), the overall Kappa statistics and other classification metrics highlight limitations in agreement and reliability, suggesting that the models require refinement to achieve clinically viable performance.

The obtained confusion matrices demonstrate greater difficulty in identifying the absence of autism, i.e., the false negative rate was lower. This finding is interesting, as it demonstrates the potential of using EEG signal processing methods with AI for ASD screening, better filtering cases in which more robust investigations. This AI-supported initial screening can be especially useful in regions with limited availability of specialized professionals.

These findings underscore the complexity of translating advanced AI techniques into robust diagnostic tools for ASD. Future studies should focus on improving feature extraction methods, enhancing the interpretability of AI models, and validating the approach on larger and more diverse and complete datasets. By continuing to refine and expand upon this integrated framework, there is substantial potential to advance the field of ASD diagnostics, ultimately contributing to earlier and more accurate interventions for individuals on the autism spectrum.

Acknowledgment(s)

This study was partially financed by the Financiadora de Estudos e Projetos – Brasil (Finep). We are also grateful to Coordenação de Aperfeiçoamento de Pessoal de Nível Superior – Brasil (CAPES), Fundação de Amparo à Ciência e Tecnologia do Estado de Pernambuco – Brasil (FACEPE), and the National Council for Scientific and Technological Development – Brasil (CNPq) for the partial financial support.

Disclosure Statement

The authors have no financial or non-financial conflict interests to declare.

References

Abdulhay, E., M. Alafeef, H. Hadoush and N. Arunkumar. (2023). A 64-channel scheme for autism detection via scaled conjugate gradient-based neural network classification of electroencephalogram ripples' complexity. *Expert Systems*, *40*(4), e13000.

Al-Qazzaz, N. K., A.A. Aldoori, A. Buniya, S.H.B.M. Ali and S.A. Ahmad. (2024). Transfer learning and hybrid deep convolutional neural networks models for autism spectrum disorder classification from EEG signals. *IEEE Access*.

Andrade, M.K., M.A. Santana, G. Moreno, I. Oliveira, J. Santos, M.C.A. Rodrigues and W.P. dos Santos. (2020). *An EEG Brain-Computer Interface to Classify Motor Imagery Signals*, pp. 83–98. Springer, Singapore.

Barbosa, V.A.F., M.A. Santana, M.K.S. Andrade, R.C.F. Lima and W.P. Santos. (2020). Deep wavelet neural networks for breast cancer early diagnosis using mammary thermographies. In: H. Das, C. Pradhan, and N. Dey (Eds.), *Deep Learning for Data Analytics: Foundations, Biomedical Applications, and Challenges* (1st Edn.). Academic Press, London.

Barbosa, V.A.F., J.C. Gomes, M.A. de Santana, E. de A. Jeniffer, R.G. de Souza, R.E. de Souza and W.P. dos Santos. (2021, Jan.). Heg.IA: An intelligent system to support diagnosis of COVID-19 based on blood tests. *Research on Biomedical Engineering*, *38*(1), 99–116.

Bouazizi, S. and H. Ltifi. (2024). Enhancing accuracy and interpretability in eeg-based medical decision making using an explainable ensemble learning framework application for stroke prediction. *Decision Support Systems*, *178*, 114126.

Cetintas, D.C., T. Tuncer and A. Cınar. (2023). Detection of autism spectrum disorder from changing of pupil diameter using multi-modal feature fusion based hybrid CNN model. *Journal of Ambient Intelligence and Humanized Computing, 14*,. 1868–5145.

Chaddad, A.Y., Wu, R. Kateb and A. Bouridane. (2023). Electroencephalography signal processing: A comprehensive review and analysis of methods and techniques. *Sensors, 23*(14), 6434.

Cruz, T.N., T.M. Cruz and W. Santos. (2018). Detection and classification of lesions in mammographies using neural networks and morphological wavelets. *IEEE Latin America Transactions, 16* (3), 926–932.

Delorme, A. and S. Makeig. (2004). EEGLAB: An open source toolbox for analysis of single-trial EEG dynamics including independent component analysis. *Journal of Neuroscience Methods, 134* (1), 9–21.

Deng, J., M. Rakibul Hasan, M. Mahmud, M. Mahbub Hasan, K. Asif Ahmed and M. Zakir Hossain. (2022). Diagnosing autism spectrum disorder using ensemble 3D-CNN: A preliminary study. In: *2022 IEEE International Conference on Image Processing (ICIP)*, pp. 3480–3484.

Deng, L. (2012). The MNIST database of handwritten digit images for machine learning research. *IEEE Signal Processing Magazine. 29*(6), 141–142.

Dickinson, A., S. Jeste and E. Milne. (2022). Electrophysiological signatures of brain aging in autism spectrum disorder. *Cortex, 148*, 139–151.

Din, Q.M. ud and A.K. Jayanthy. (2022). Wavelet scattering transform and deep learning networks based autism spectrum disorder identification using EEG signals. *Traitement du Signal, 39*(6), 2069.

Eaton, J.W., D. Bateman, S. Hauberg and R. Wehbring. (2019). *GNU Octave Version 5.1.0 Manual: A High-level Interactive Language for Numerical Computations*. URL https://www.gnu.org/software/octave/doc/v5.1.0/.

Gomes, J.C., V.A.d.F. Barbosa, M.A. Santana, J. Bandeira, M.J.S. Valença, R.E. de Souza, A.M. Ismael and W.P. dos Santos. (2020). IKONOS: An intelligent tool to support diagnosis of COVID-19 by texture analysis of x-ray images. *Research on Biomedical Engineering*, 1–14.

Hus, Y. and O. Segal. (2021). Challenges surrounding the diagnosis of autism in children. *Neuropsychiatric Disease and Treatment,* 3509–3529.

Kang, J., X. Han, J. Song, Z. Niu and X. Li. (2020). The identification of children with autism spectrum disorder by SVM approach on EEG and eye-tracking data. *Computers in Biology and Medicine, 120*, 103722.

Kashef, R. (2022). ECNN: Enhanced convolutional neural network for efficient diagnosis of autism spectrum disorder. *Cognitive Systems Research, 71*, 41–49. ISSN 1389-0417. https://www.sciencedirect.com/science/article/pii/S1389041721000759.

Kemp, B. and J. Olivan. (2003). European data format 'plus' (edf+), an EDF alike standard format for the exchange of physiological data. *Clinical Neurophysiology, 114*(9), 1755–1761.

Lang, S., F. Bravo-Marquez, C. Beckham, M. Hall and E. Frank. (2019). Wekadeeplearning4j: A deep learning package for Weka based on deeplearning4j. *Knowledge-Based Systems, 178*, 48–50.

LeCun, Y., L. Bottou, Y. Bengio and P. Haffner. (1998). Gradient-based learning applied to document recognition. *Proceedings of the IEEE, 86*(11), 2278–2324.

Mallat, S.G. (1989). Multifrequency channel decompositions of images and wavelet models. *IEEE Trans. Acoustics, Speech, and Signal Processing*, *37*(12), 2091–2110.

Maor, E. (2019). *The Pythagorean Theorem: A 4,000-Year History* (Vol. 65). Princeton Science Library.

Oliver, E., J. Ruiz, S. She and J. Wang. (2006). The software architecture of the GIMP. *Scribd.*

Oliveira, A.P.S., M.A. Santana, M.K.S. Andrade, J.C. Gomes, M.C. Rodrigues and W.P. dos Santos. (2020). Early diagnosis of parkinson's disease using EEG, machine learning and partial directed coherence. *Research on Biomedical Engineering*, *36*(3), 311–331.

Oostenveld, R. and P. Praamstra. (2001). The five percent electrode system for high-resolution EEG and ERP measurements. *Clinical Neurophysiology*, *112*(4), 713–719.

Peketi, S. and S.B. Dhok. (2023). Machine learning enabled p300 classifier for autism spectrum disorder using adaptive signal decomposition. *Brain Sciences*, *13*(2), 315.

Sai, K.V.K., R.T. Krishna, K. Radha, Rao, D. Venkata and A. Muneera. (2024). Automated ASD detection in children from raw speech using customized STFT-CNN model. *International Journal of Speech Technology*, 1572–8110.

Santana, M.A., J.C. Gomes, G.M. de Souza, A. Suarez, A.S. Torcate, F.S. Fonseca, G.M.M. Moreno and W.P. dos Santos. (2020a). Reconhecimento automático de emoções a partir de sinais multimodais e inteligência artificial. *Anais do IV Simpósio de Inovação em Engenharia Biomédica-SABIO 2020*, p. 43.

Santana, M.A., J.M.S. Pereira, R.C.F. Lima and W.P. Santos. (2020b). Breast lesions classification in frontal thermographic images using intelligent systems and moments of Haralick and Zernike. In: W.P. dos Santos, M.A. de Santana and W.W.A. da Silva (Eds.), *Understanding a Cancer Diagnosis* (1st Edn.), pp. 65–80. Nova Science, New York.

Santana, M.A., J.M.S. Pereira, F.L. Silva, N.M. Lima, F.N. Sousa, G.M.S. Arruda, R.C.F.d. Lima, W.W.A. Silva and W.P. Santos. (2018). Breast cancer diagnosis based on mammary thermography and extreme learning machines. *Research on Biomedical Engineering*, *34*, 45–53. ISSN 2446-4740.

Santana, M.A., F.S. Fonseca, A.S. Torcate and W.P. dos Santos. (2023). Emotion recognition from multimodal data: A machine learning approach combining classical and hybrid deep architectures. *Research on Biomedical Engineering*, *39*(3), 613–638.

Santana, M.A. (2023). *Arquiteturas de redes profundas para interfaces musicais humano-máquina para reconhecimento de emoções em sinais eletroencefalográficos e de voz como apoio à musicoterapia*. PhD Thesis, Universidade de Pernambuco, Recife, Brazil. URL 10.13140/RG.2.2.22104.30725.

Santana, M.A. and W.P. Santos. (2024). Therapies customization by emotion recognition in biosignals, 16(Especial). ResearchGate.

Van Rossum, G. and F.L. Drake. (2009). *Python 3 Reference Manual*. CreateSpace, Scotts Valley, CA. ISBN 1441412697.

Witten, I.H. and E. Frank. (2005). *Data Mining: Practical Machine Learning Tools and Technique*. Morgan Kaufmann Publishers, San Francisco, CA, USA.

World Health Organization (WHO). (2023). Autism. Accessed December, 2024. https://www.who.int/news-room/fact-sheets/detail/autism-spectrum-disorders.

7 Advances in Differential Diagnosis of ASD
EEG Electrode Reduction with Machine Learning

Flávio Secco Fonseca[1*], Maria Vitória Soares Muniz[2], Ana Beatriz de Souza Sampaio[2], Maria Luísa Mendes de Siqueira Passos[2] and Wellington Pinheiro dos Santos[2]

Autism Spectrum Disorder (ASD) arises from difficulties with communication and social interaction. This context creates an urgent need for more effective differential diagnostics. This chapter evaluates electrode reduction in EEG examinations to improve ASD diagnosis with machine learning methods. We use the Sheffield Public Database, which includes EEG signals from individuals with ASD. Our methodology applies an innovative interpolation formula to address absent signals. Particle swarm optimization (PSO) algorithms select the most relevant features. This approach reduces the initial number of electrodes from 64 to 17. We also implement a second approach that retains only 9 electrodes from the front-central and front-temporal regions. One classifier achieves accuracy above 99%. This result shows the presence of discriminative EEG patterns related to ASD. Our work increases the efficiency and accessibility of ASD diagnosis. Early interventions lead to better prognoses and quality of life. This approach also improves processes in the healthcare system.

1. Introduction

Autism Spectrum Disorder (ASD) is a neurological developmental condition. It involves difficulties with communication and social interaction. It also features repetitive and restrictive behaviors (American Psychiatric Association, 2013). Researchers now view ASD as a spectrum because of its broad range of manifestations. Some definitions emphasize comprehensive perspectives on autism. Others focus on detailed diagnoses within neurodevelopmental disorders (Lord et al., 2018).

ASD affects individuals and families over the long term. It requires consistent support and specific treatment resources (Lord et al., 2020).

1 Universidade de Pernambuco, Pernambuco, Brazil.
2 Universidade Federal de Pernambuco, Pernambuco, Brazil.
* Corresponding author: fsf2@ecomp.poli.br.

DOI: 10.1201/9781003531418-7

Clinicians classify ASD into three support levels. Level 1 demands some assistance. Level 2 calls for more substantial help. Level 3 involves very intensive intervention (Kulage et al., 2014; Volkmar and Reichow, 2013; Kulage et al., 2020). Global records revealed about 60.38 million new cases in 2019. By that period, around 283.25 million cases had reached formal diagnosis (Li et al., 2021).

Signs of ASD often emerge between 12–24 months of age. Interventions before age two can influence brain development in children with ASD (Yoo, 2016). However, early diagnosis does not always happen at the ideal time. It requires a multidisciplinary team of professionals. These teams include speech therapists, psychologists, pediatricians, psychiatrists, and occupational therapists (Saleem et al., 2021; Rani et al., 2022). This situation drives the need for new technologies. Faster and simpler diagnostic methods lead to earlier, more accurate, and more accessible autism diagnoses for all.

In this context, many researchers have explored alternative methods that involve electroencephalogram (EEG) signals. EEG records brain electrical activity through electrodes that scientists place on the scalp. It detects impulses arising from neuronal communication (de Almeida et al., 2021). Meanwhile, machine learning has yielded diagnostic support tools (Heinsfeld et al., 2018; Kho datars et al., 2021). This field belongs to artificial intelligence. It relies on algorithms and statistical models that detect patterns and execute specific tasks without explicit instructions for each function (Pag nozzi et al., 2018).

This chapter introduces a new approach for the differential diagnosis of ASD. It merges machine learning algorithms with EEG systems that use few electrodes or low-density configurations. We also propose a method that addresses missing signals, a common obstacle in EEG databases. The next sections present the theoretical foundation, methodology, results, and conclusions.

2. Theoretical Foundation

This chapter requires essential knowledge of machine learning and electroencephalography (EEG). First, we introduce core ideas from machine learning, with special attention to its supervised subfield. Then, we present basic concepts related to EEG.

2.1 Machine Learning

Machine learning is a major discipline within artificial intelligence (AI). It involves algorithms that detect patterns, classify datasets, and predict outcomes from existing information (Tarca et al., 2007). These algorithms enable computers to emulate human reasoning and adapt to previous examples with minimal human guidance (Mahadevkar et al., 2022). Supervised learning relies on labeled input/output pairs. Models trained under this approach anticipate future results based on historical data. Common supervised algorithms include Bayesian Networks, Naive Bayes, Random Tree, Random Forest, and Support Vector Machines (SVMs). Each one addresses specific applications and offers distinct strengths.

Bayesian Networks rely on Bayes' theorem. They operate as graphical models for probabilistic inference (Zhao et al., 2011; Yuan et al., 2020) and outline joint probability distributions over time (Wu et al., 2015). Each network has a qualitative section, which forms a directed acyclic graph (DAG), and a quantitative section, which defines conditional probabilities (Darwiche, 2008).

Bayesian decision theorem states that a Bayesian classifier picks the class with the highest membership probability for a test instance. The algorithm uses training data to estimate prior and posterior distributions. It also relies on attribute relationships to model these posterior distributions (Kim and Lee, 2022). This structure grants Bayesian networks a strong advantage under uncertain data. It draws on the principles of probability theory (Atienza et al., 2022).

Among Bayesian classifiers, Naive Bayes stands out for its simple structure. It treats every attribute in the training data as conditionally independent and equally important for classification. It then computes probabilities by counting frequencies and value combinations in the dataset (Dimitoglou et al., 2012).

A decision tree is a graph with one root node and branches (directed links) to child nodes, which may branch out further (Cañete Sifuentes et al., 2021). Random Tree is a specific decision tree model that selects a subset of attributes at random (Niranjan et al., 2018). It constructs a subset of possible trees, then picks one with equal probability (Shubho et al., 2019).

Random Forest relies on an ensemble of tree-based models. It merges the outputs of multiple decision trees to classify or regress by majority vote or by averaging results (Chen et al., 2024). The algorithm uses random data samples to form each tree and improves accuracy through diverse perspectives (Dong et al., 2019). Researchers have shown that Random Forest excels at EEG signal classification. It thus serves as a valuable tool for diagnosing ASD (Kong et al., 2023; Kumar et al., 2023).

SVMs, introduced by Vapnik, are supervised learning methods for classification, regression, and ranking (Chamasemani and Singh, 2011). They excel at separating data into two groups in a high-dimensional feature space. The SVM algorithm identifies an optimal hyperplane in N-dimensional space that classifies data points with maximum margin (Sari et al., 2011). The closest vector to this hyperplane, called the Support Vector, defines the separation margin (PD and Haryoko, 2022). SVM also delivers high accuracy when classifying EEG signals and is considered one of the most effective classifiers in brain-computer interfaces (Antunes et al., 2023; Hao et al., 2023; Patil and Patil, 2023).

2.2 EEG

Our focus on electrode reduction requires knowledge of EEG methods, types, and patterns. EEG records electrical signals generated by brain cells through electrodes. The 10–20 system by Malmivuo and Plonsey (1995) is the standard for electrode placement. Its name refers to the electrode position and the underlying cerebral cortex line. The "10" or "20" indicates the percentage distance between electrodes along the front-back and left-right axes (UFU line).

3. Methodology

This chapter's methodology follows a clear sequence. We first conduct an exploratory analysis of the database for each experiment. We then outline the preprocessing steps that the database undergoes. We next describe the complete database and alternative approaches. Finally, we present each configuration for classification and explain the chosen evaluation metrics.

3.1 Database

This study uses Dataset 1 from the Sheffield database (Dickinson et al., 2022). It includes EEG signals from 56 individuals. Researchers collected these signals with the Biosemi Active Two EEG system. Participants were 18–68 years old. Each session lasted 150 seconds, with eyes closed at rest and during visual stimulation. The band-pass filter ranged from 0.01 to 140 Hz, and Cz served as the reference channel.

Most participants used a 64-sensor setup (Dickinson et al., 2022). Some used a 128-sensor arrangement (Oostenveld and Praamstra, 2001). Researchers modified the 128-sensor data to match the 64-sensor version, ensuring consistency across groups. EEGLAB (Delorme and Makeig, 2004) applies a 1 Hz transition band and passband margin to filter the continuous data. The final data has a 512 Hz sampling rate. Researchers removed corrupted or anomalous segments before releasing the dataset.

We observed several issues during the exploratory analysis. Missing electrodes posed the main challenge (Figure 1). They represent 11.51% of the total data. The dataframe includes 64 columns (electrodes) and 81,921 rows, leading to 262,918,054 data points. Missing signals appear in 53% of the control group and 47% of the autistic group. Figure 1 shows that most files lack signals for zero to seven electrodes. Only one individual has all 64 electrodes with complete signals.

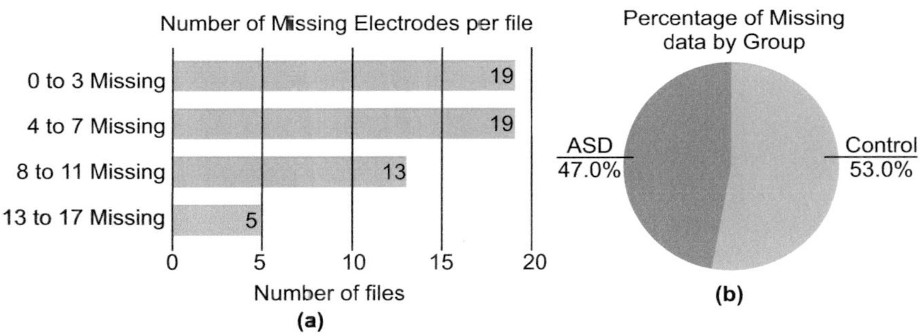

Fig. 1 Missing data graphs. (a) A bar graph shows how many electrodes are missing for each individual. (b) A pie chart shows the percentage of missing data in the control and ASD groups.

We conducted a survey of missing electrodes in several brain regions (Duan et al., 2020). These regions include the frontal, central, temporal, parietal, and occipital areas. Figure 2 shows that the central region contains the largest number of missing electrodes, followed by the frontal region. The frontal-polar region has the fewest missing data. It only involves the FPZ electrode.

Missing electrodes often appear in EEG databases because of interference or involuntary movements. These absent signals create data gaps. They produce incomplete representations of brain activity. This situation hinders the analysis of results. The lack of a standardized electrode placement system also poses a noticeable issue in this database. Variations in exact electrode locations affect measurement accuracy and alter interpretations of brain activity patterns. High-electrode density systems add another challenge. They offer comprehensive coverage and improved spatial resolution, but they also generate large data volumes. This volume can exceed computational resources and complicate the identification of brain patterns.

3.2 Pre Processing

We converted the original .set and .fdt files from the Sheffield dataset to .edf and .csv formats to enable machine learning applications. The European Data Format (.edf) is a standard for sharing EEG and polysomnography data across different equipment and laboratories, but it provides limited functionality for other analyses (Kemp and Olivan, 2003). We used an additional conversion to .csv format to simplify data manipulation. We carried out all conversion

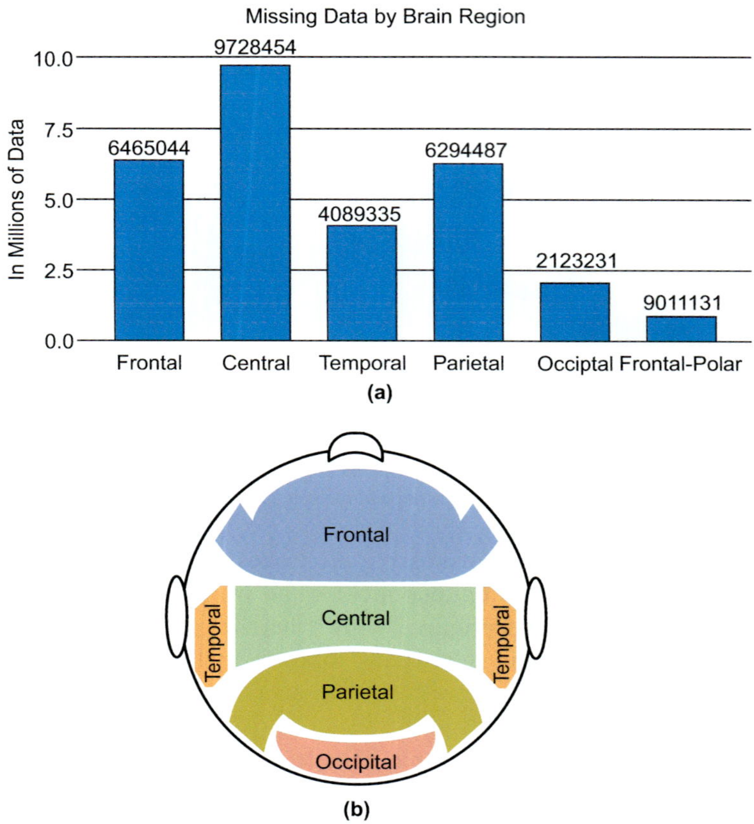

Fig. 2 (a) Graphs of missing data by brain region. (b) Map of cerebral cortex regions.

steps and data processing with Python 3.11.1 (Van Rossum and Drake, 2009). Figure 3 shows a diagram of this entire conversion process and the data processing flow.

In the previous section, we identified missing data in the database as the main issue. We adopt the Inverse Distance Weighting (IDW) method to solve this problem. Many researchers consider IDW effective for spatial interpolation, especially in geoscientific and geographic data (Li and Wang, 2013). Studies also report its success in estimating missing values on cortical surfaces (Vandekar et al., 2015).

IDW is a deterministic method that uses a linear combination of known samples to estimate unknown points. It assumes that closer samples better represent missing values than distant ones (Chen and Liu, 2012; Oktavia et al., 2016). We adopt a modified version of IDW to reduce computational cost

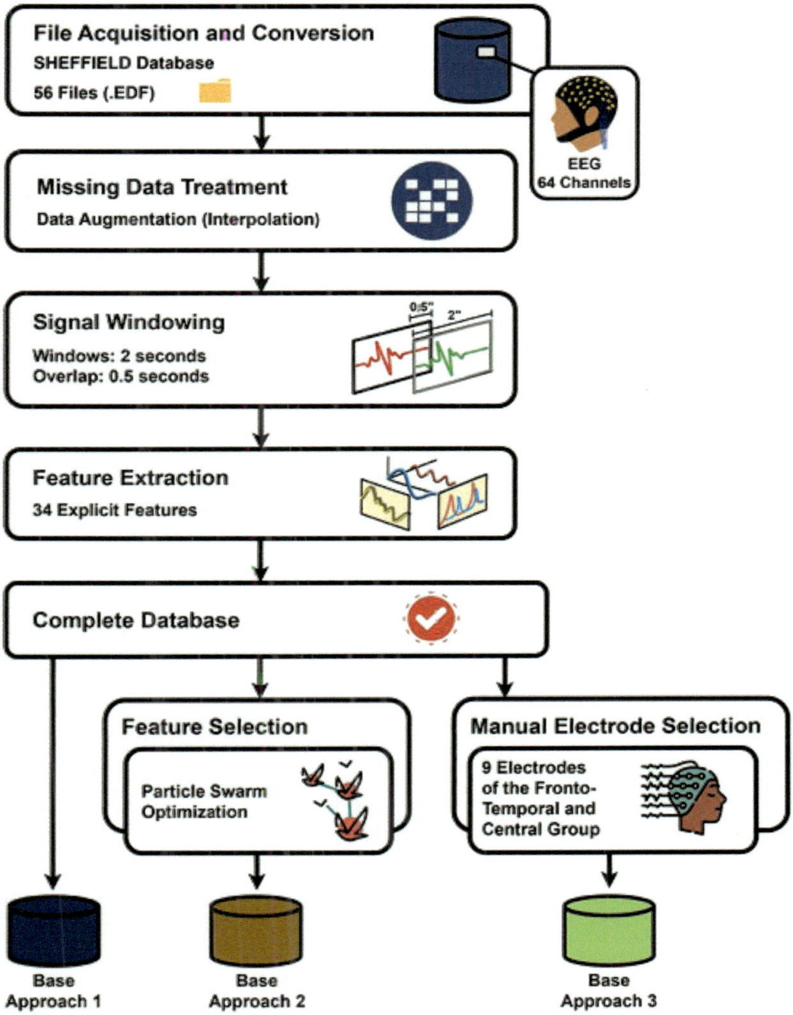

Fig. 3 Database pre-processing steps. Treatment of missing signals and windowing; Feature extraction; Feature selection; Division of the dataset into a Training/Validation and Test set; Tuning hyperparameters of classification models.

and avoid division-by-zero errors. Instead of using the inverse of distance, we apply a negative exponential function (Equation 1). In this interpolation context, "*Pj*" refers to the missing channel, and "*Pi*" indicates available channels. This approach aims to minimize error propagation through a simple and efficient interpolation.

$$P_j = \frac{\sum_{i=1}^{m} P_i e^{-d_{ij}}}{\sum_{i=1}^{m} e^{-d_{ij}}} \quad ...(1)$$

We implement the IDW method by first calculating the coordinates of the 64 electrodes. We rely on GIMP software (version 2.10.34) for this step (Oliver et al., 2006). We then apply Equation 2 to compute the distance between two electrodes. In that equation, "*a*" and "*b*" represent the points, and "*x*1"/"*y*1" and "*x*2"/"*y*2" indicate the coordinates for "*a*" and "*b* ", respectively.

$$d_{ab} = \sqrt{(x_2 - x_1)^2 + (y_2 - y_1)^2} \quad ...(2)$$

After the interpolation step, we use GNU Octave Version 8.2.0 (Eaton et al., 2023) to segment the data into windows and extract features. Each window produces 34 attributes, as shown in Figure 4. These attributes include statistical measures such as mean, variance, standard deviation, square root of the mean, mean amplitude variation, absolute deviation of the difference, integrated absolute value, logarithm detector, simple quadratic integral, mean absolute value, mean logarithmic kernel, skewness, kurtosis, maximum amplitude, and 3rd, 4th, and 5th order moments.

We also extract time-frequency domain attributes, including waveform length, zero crossing, signal slope variations, Hjorth parameters (activity, mobility, complexity), mean frequency, median frequency, mean power, peak frequency, power spectrum ratio, total power, central frequency variance, Shannon entropy, and 1st, 2nd, and 3rd order spectral moments. Previous studies on EEG and peripheral physiological signals confirm the effectiveness of these attributes (de Santana et al., 2023). We work with 64 electrodes and obtain 2,176 attributes. Each window spans 2 seconds, with a 0.5-second overlap and a 512 Hz sampling rate.

3.3 Applied Approaches

We now describe the approaches used in this chapter. We first validate the interpolation method. We then introduce the initial approach with the complete database. Next, we apply feature selection through Particle Swarm Optimization (PSO). Finally, we present an approach that uses nine manually selected electrodes.

3.3.1 Validation of the Interpolation Method

We aim to confirm the effectiveness of the interpolation method. We choose two pairs of electrodes, CP1/CP2 and FC1/FC2, because they appear most

Parameter	*Equation*	*Parameter*	*Equation*
Mean (m)	$\mu = \frac{1}{N}\sum_{n=1}^{N} x_n$	**Waveform length**	$WL = \sum_{n=1}^{N-1} \lvert x_{n+1} - x_n \rvert$
Variance	$\text{var} = \frac{1}{N-1}\sum_{n=1}^{N}(x_n - \mu)^2$	**Zero crossing**	$ZC = \sum_{n=1}^{N-1} [sgn(x_n \times x_{n+1}) \cap \lvert x_n - x_{n+1}\rvert \geq \text{threshold}]$ $sgn(x) = \begin{cases} 1, if\ x \geq \text{threshold} \\ 0, \quad \text{otherwise} \end{cases}$
Standard deviation (s)	$\sigma = \sqrt{\frac{1}{N-1}\sum_{n=1}^{N}\lvert x_n - \mu \rvert^2}$	**Slope Sign Changes**	$SSC = \sum_{n=1}^{N-1} [f(x_n - x_{n-1}) \times (x_n - x_{n+1})]$ $f(x) = \begin{cases} 1, if\ x \geq \text{threshold} \\ 0, \quad \text{otherwise} \end{cases}$
Root mean square	$RMS = \sqrt{\frac{\sum_{n=1}^{N}(x_n)^2}{N}}$	**Hjorth parameter activity**	$Hjorth_{activity} = \frac{1}{N-1}\sum_{n=1}^{N}(x_n - \mu)^2$
Average Amplitude Changes	$ACC = \frac{1}{N}\left(\sum_{n=1}^{N}\left\lvert\frac{dx(t)}{dt}\right\rvert\right)$	**Hjorth parameter mobility**	$Hjorth_{mobility} = \sqrt{\frac{\frac{\text{var}(dx(t))}{dt}}{\text{var}(x(t))}}$
Difference Absolute Deviation	$DASDV = \sqrt{\frac{1}{N}\sum_{n=1}^{N}\left(\frac{dx(t)}{dt}\right)^2}$	**Hjorth parameter complexity**	$Hjorth_{complexity} = \frac{Hjorth_{mobility}\left(\frac{dx(t)}{dt}\right)}{Hjorth_{mobility}\ (x(t))}$

Contd.

Fig. 4 *Contd.*

Parameter	*Equation*	*Parameter*	*Equation*
Integrated Absolute Value	$IAV = \sum_{n=1}^{N} x_n$	**Mean frequency**	$MNF = \frac{\sum_{j=1}^{M} f_j P_j}{\sum_{j=1}^{M} P_j}$ Where f_j, P_j are the frequencies and power of the spectrum, respectively, and M is the length of the frequencies
Logarithm Detector	$LOGD = e^{\left(\frac{1}{N}\sum_{n=1}^{N} \log(\lvert x_n \rvert)\right)}$	**Median frequency**	$MDF = \frac{1}{2}\sum_{j=1}^{M} P_j$
Simple Square Integral	$\mathrm{SSI} = \sum_{n=1}^{N} {x_n}^2$	**Mean power**	$MNP = \sum_{j=1}^{M} \frac{P_j}{M}$
Mean Absolute Value	$\mathrm{MAV} = \frac{1}{N}\sum_{n=1}^{N} \lvert x_n \rvert$	**Peak frequency**	$PKF = \max(P_j)$
Mean Logarithm Kernel	$\mathrm{MLOGK} = \frac{1}{N}\left\lvert \sum_{n=1}^{N} x_n \right\rvert$	**Power Spectrum ratio**	$PSR = \frac{PKF}{\sum_{j=1}^{M} P_j}$
Skewness (s)	$s = \frac{\frac{1}{N}\sum_{n=1}^{N} (x_n - \mu)^3}{\sigma^2}$	**Total Power**	$TP = \sum_{j=1}^{M} P_j$

Contd.

Fig. 4 *Contd.*

Parameter	*Equation*	*Parameter*	*Equation*
Kurtosis	$\text{kurt} = \frac{\frac{1}{N}\sum_{n=1}^{N}(x_n - \mu)^4}{\sigma^4}$	**First Spectral Moment**	$SM1 = \sum_{j=1}^{M} f_j P_j$
Maximum Amplitude	$MAX = \max(x_n)$	**Second Spectral Moment**	$SM2 = \sum_{j-1}^{M} f_j^{\,2} P_j$
Third Moment	$M3 = \left\lvert \frac{1}{N}\sum_{n-1}^{N}(x_n)^3 \right\rvert$	**Third Spectral Moment**	$SM3 = \sum_{j=1}^{M} f_j^{\,3} P_j$
Fourth Moment	$M4 = \left\lvert \frac{1}{N}\sum_{n-1}^{N}(x_n)^4 \right\rvert$	**Variance of Central Frequency**	$VCF - \frac{SM2}{TP} - \left(\frac{SM1}{TP}\right)^2$
Fifth Moment	$M5 = \left\lvert \frac{1}{N}\sum_{n-1}^{N}(x_n)^5 \right\rvert$	**Shannon's entropy**	$E = -\sum_i S_i^2 \log(S_i^2)$, where S is the signal

Fig. 4 Table with 34 explicit attributes, extracted from the signals.

frequently among the 56 individuals in the database. CP1 lacks signals in two individuals with ASD, while CP2 is missing signals in four individuals. FC1 and FC2 each have three individuals without signals. We apply the interpolation method to these four electrodes to minimize its impact on final classification.

Figure 5 outlines the three steps that validate the interpolation approach for treating missing signals. We first test classifiers on the dataset with all four electrodes. We then analyze each pair, FC and CP, on its own.

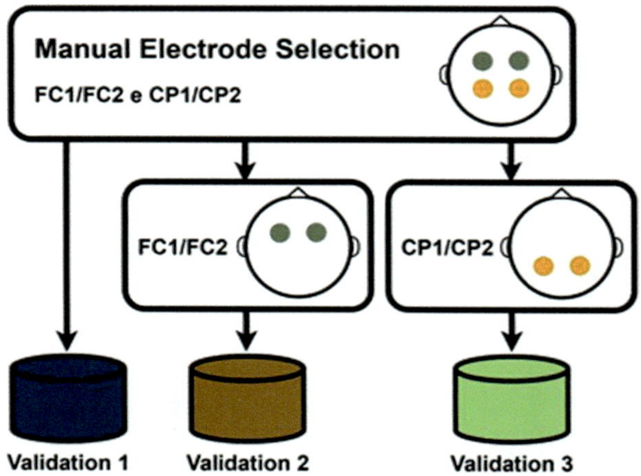

Fig. 5 Diagram summarizing the approaches explored to validate the effectiveness of the interpolation method. Approach with the 4 electrodes of the FC and CP group. Approach with the FC1 and FC2 electrodes. Approach with the CP1 and CP2 electrodes.

3.3.2 Complete Base

In this approach, we select the complete dataset with all 64 electrodes (63 + reference electrode). Each electrode has 34 explicit attributes, totaling 2,142 attributes per individual. We then apply two strategies. First, we use PSO for feature selection. Next, we manually choose 9 electrodes from the fronto-central region.

3.3.3 PSO

We run the PSO algorithm on the original dataset to select attributes. The algorithm picks 686 attributes out of the 2,142 available in the complete dataset. These attributes span all 64 electrodes.

3.3.4 9 (Nine) Electrodes

We also select 9 electrodes after examining previous scientific studies. Researchers observed a marked drop in brain activation in the left frontotemporal region of individuals with ASD compared to neurotypical controls. This drop appears during social and non-social tasks, reflecting the role of this region in key cognitive functions that ASD often impairs. We choose FT7, FC5, FC3, FC1, FCz, FC2, FC4, FC6, and FT8 (Figure 6). These electrodes cover frontal and central cortical areas linked to attention, sensory perception, decision-making, and social processing. Focusing on these locations captures crucial electrical signals linked to cognitive and sensory issues in ASD. This selection produces a dataset with 306 attributes per class ("With ASD" and "Without ASD"). It offers a concise set of signals for machine learning algorithms that diagnose ASD from EEG data.

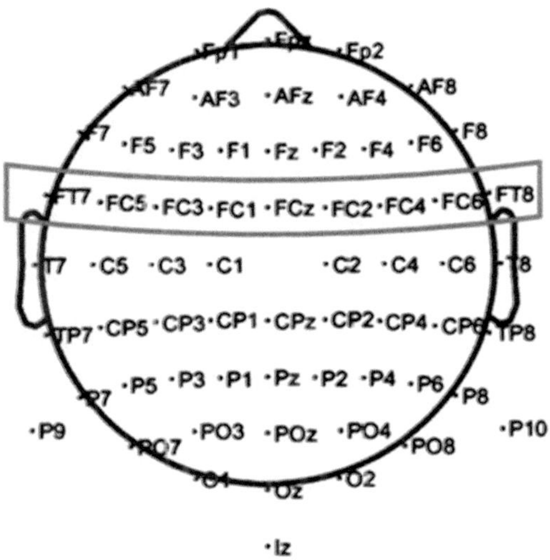

Fig. 6 Map of the 64 electrodes, with 9 electrodes from the FT and FC groups highlighted.

3.4 Classification

We processed the data from each approach and then trained, validated, and tested multiple classifiers. These classifiers included Bayes Net, Naive Bayes, Random Tree, Random Forest (with 10, 100, and 500 trees), and SVMs with linear kernels, polynomial kernels (degrees 2 and 3), and RBF kernels (Gamma 0.1, 0.2, and 0.5).

We used the Waikato Environment for Knowledge Analysis (WEKA), version 3.9.6 (Eibe et al., 2016; Hall et al., 2009). We split each dataset into

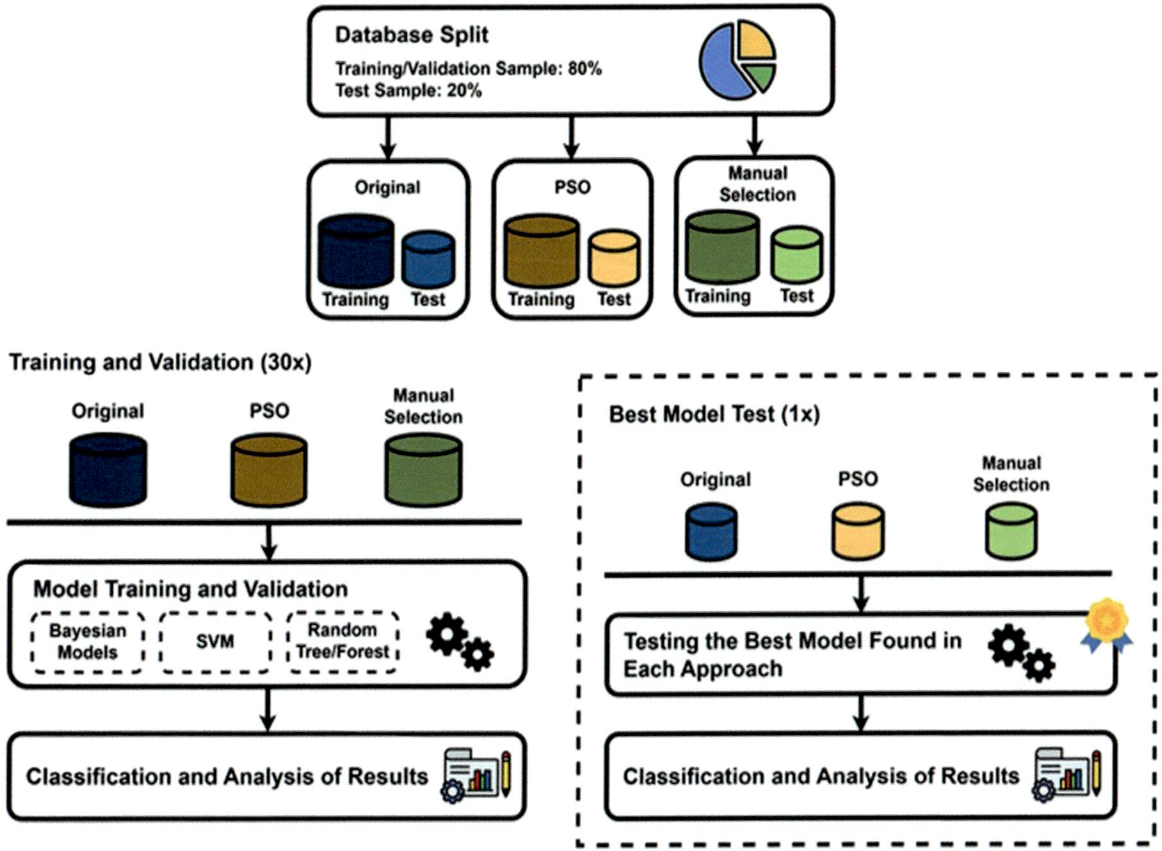

Fig. 7 Diagram of the classification steps. Division of the base into training and testing. Trained and tested models.

80% for training and 20% for testing. We ran 30 experiment repetitions and used 10-fold cross-validation to boost statistical confidence. Cross-validation avoids overly optimistic results and encourages model generalization by training on different data subsets and averaging the outcomes (Calomino et al., 2024). Figure 7 shows a diagram of these steps.

3.5 Metrics

We use five metrics to evaluate the models in both the training and testing phases: accuracy, Kappa, sensitivity, specificity, and the area under the ROC (Receiver Operating Characteristic) curve. Accuracy shows how well the classifier predicts the correct class of each instance, relying on true positive and true negative rates. The Kappa index measures the agreement between the data and the classification and reflects the proportion of agreement adjusted by chance (Fonseca et al., 2022). Its maximum value is 1. Values above 0.75 indicate excellent agreement, while values between 0.40 and 0.75 suggest medium agreement (de Menezes et al., 2023).

Sensitivity (or recall) measures the probability that positive classifications match the actual positives (Nunes et al., 2024). Specificity measures the classifier's ability to identify healthy patients as negative, thus focusing on the rate of true negatives (Gomes et al., 2023). The ROC curve plots the false positive rate on the x-axis and the true positive rate (sensitivity) on the y-axis. It offers a probabilistic view of the model's predictive power, and the area under the curve reflects this probability. Table 1 shows these metrics and their mathematical expressions (de Santana et al., 2023).

4. Results

This section presents this study's results. First, it examines how the IDW interpolation method performs. Next, it analyzes the complete dataset with all 64 electrodes, which serves as a strong reference. To optimize and reduce the dimensionality, it then applies PSO and manually selects 9 electrodes. For each classifier, it calculates mean and standard deviation scores for each metric over 30 training runs. It also tests the best models from each dataset to identify the most effective techniques. This procedure highlights the strongest methods and guides future work.

4.1 Validation of the Method

This validation begins with the combined CP1/2 and FC1/2 electrodes. Table 2 shows the results for all classifiers.

Table 1 The metrics used and their formulas TP, TN, FP, and FN represent the quantity of True Positives, True Negatives, False Positives and False Negatives, respectively. TPR and FPR represent the True Positive Rate and False Positive Rate, respectively.

Metric	*Mathematical expression*
Accuracy	$ACC = \frac{TP + TN}{TP + TN + FP + FN}$
Kappa	$K = \frac{(ro - re)}{(1 - re)}$
	where ÿo is the observed agreement rate and ye is the expected agreement rate, given by:
	$\ddot{y}e = \frac{(TP + FP)\,(TP + FN) + (FN + TN)\,(FP + FN)}{TP + FP + FN + TN}$
Sensitivity	$Sens = \frac{TP}{TP + FP}$
Specificity	$Esp = \frac{TN}{TN + FP}$
Area under the ROC curve AUC = TPR d(FPR)	

Tree-based symbolic models excel. Random decision forests with 10, 100, and 500 trees exceed 95% accuracy, surpass 96% average sensitivity, and remain above 94% average specificity. Their symbolic nature also facilitates interpretation. Bayesian models struggle. Naive Bayes achieves only 62% accuracy and the lowest Kappa, sensitivity, specificity, and area under the ROC curve.

Table 3 presents the results for the CP electrode group. Performance drops by about 5–10% compared to the four-electrode approach. The ranking of best and worst models remains the same. Random Forest continues to top the list, with minimal variance across different tree configurations. Bayesian models still rank lowest. Support Vector Machines deliver intermediate results, ranging from 75 to 90% accuracy, depending on the chosen configuration.

Table 4 shows the results when using only the FC electrodes. This experiment reveals no major differences compared to the classification with the CP group. The average and standard deviation of each metric follow a similar pattern. Bayes Net stands out with a noticeable increase in accuracy, Kappa index, and specificity.

These three approaches confirm the viability of classifying individuals on the autism spectrum. Yet, they also suggest that more electrodes could boost the model's sensitivity. Another hypothesis emerges around the chosen cortical region, reinforcing the idea that the FC electrodes may play the primary role in the diagnostic process.

Table 2 Training and validation results using the CP and FC group electrodes combined.

Classifier		*Accuracy (%)*	*Kappa Index*	*Sensitivity*	*Specificity*	*AUC*
Bayes Net	-	71.57 ± 2.08	0.44 ± 0.04	0.78 ± 0.03	0.66 ± 0.03	0.82 ± 0.02
Naive Bayes	-	62.30 ± 2.04	0.22 ± 0.05	0.34 ± 0.03	0.86 ± 0.02	0.70 ± 0.02
Random Tree	-	89.48 ± 1.70	0.79 ± 0.03	0.89 ± 0.03	0.90 ± 0.02	0.89 ± 0.02
Rdm Forest	10	95.21 ± 1.12	0.90 ± 0.02	0.96 ± 0.01	0.94 ± 0.02	0.99 ± 0.00
	100	96.80 ± 0.92	0.94 ± 0.02	0.97 ± 0.01	0.97 ± 0.01	1.00 ± 0.00
	500	96.90 ± 0.90	0.94 ± 0.02	0.97 ± 0.01	0.97 ± 0.01	1.00 ± 0.00
SVM	Poly (Linear)	75.92 ± 2.10	0.52 ± 0.04	0.73 ± 0.03	0.78 ± 0.03	0.76 ± 0.02
	Poli 2	89.80 ± 1.46	0.79 ± 0.03	0.88 ±0.03	0.91 ± 0.02	0.90 ± 0.01
	Poli 3	93.68 ± 1.21	0.87 ± 0.02	0.93 ± 0.02	0.94 ± 0.02	0.94 ± 0.01
SVM	RBF 0.5	90.85 ± 1.35	0.82 ± 0.03	0.90 ± 0.02	0.92 ± 0.02	0.91 ± 0.01
	RBF 0.2	83.17 ± 1.94	0.66 ± 0.04	0.83 ± 0.03	0.84 ± 0.03	0.83 ± 0.02
	RBF 0.1	77.65 ± 2.03	0.55 ± 0.04	0.77 ± 0.03	0.77 ± 0.03	0.78 ± 0.02

Table 3 Training and validation results using the CP group electrodes.

Classifier		*Accuracy (%)*	*Kappa Index*	*Sensitivity*	*Specificity*	*AUC*
Bayes Net	-	66.19 ± 2.15	0.33 ± 0.04	0.77 ± 0.03	0.57 ± 0.03	0.76 ± 0.02
Naive Bayes	-	56.57 ± 2.04	0.1 ± 0.04	0.35 ± 0.04	0.75 ± 0.03	0.64 ± 0.02
Random Tree	-	83.31 ± 1.95	0.66 ± 0.04	0.82 ± 0.03	0.84 ± 0.03	0.83 ± 0.02
Rdm Forest	10	89.08 ± 1.53	0.78 ± 0.03	0.92 ± 0.02	0.87 ± 0.02	0.96 ± 0.01
	100	91.1 ± 1.31	0.82 ± 0.03	0.93 ± 0.02	0.9 ± 0.02	0.97 ± 0.01
	500	91.25 ± 1.36	0.82 ± 0.03	0.93 ± 0.02	0.9 ± 0.02	0.97 ± 0.01
SVM	Poly (Linear)	67.27 ± 2.25	0.34 ± 0.05	0.62 ± 0.04	0.72 ± 0.03	0.67 ± 0.02
	Poli 2	77.72 ± 2.13	0.55 ± 0.04	0.79 ± 0.03	0.77 ± 0.03	0.78 ± 0.02
	Poli 3	84.32 ± 1.67	0.69 ± 0.03	0.85 ± 0.03	0.84 ± 0.02	0.84 ± 0.02
SVM	RBF 0.1	67.71 ± 2.16	0.35 ± 0.04	0.63 ± 0.04	0.72 ± 0.03	0.67 ± 0.02
	RBF 0.2	79.18 ± 2.20	0.40 ± 0.04	0.71 ± 0.03	0.72 ± 0.03	0.70 ± 0.02
	RBF 0.5	79.59 ± 2.10	0.59 ± 0.04	0.84 ± 0.03	0.76 ± 0.03	0.80 ± 0.02

Table 4 Training and validation results using the FC group electrodes.

Classifier		*Accuracy (%)*	*Kappa Index*	*Sensitivity*	*Specificity*	*AUC*
Bayes Net	-	72.45 ± 2.13	0.45 ± 0.04	0.79 ± 0.03	0.67 ± 0.03	0.80 ± 0.02
Naive Bayes	-	59.14 ± 1.40	0.17 ± 0.03	0.22 ± 0.03	0.95 ± 0.02	0.69 ± 0.02
Random Tree	-	82.99 ± 1.96	0.66 ± 0.04	0.83 ± 0.03	0.83 ± 0.03	0.83 ± 0.02
Rdm Forest	10	88.72 ± 1.46	0.77 ± 0.03	0.91 ± 0.02	0.86 ± 0.02	0.96 ± 0.01
	100	90.81 ± 1.42	0.82 ± 0.03	0.91 ± 0.02	0.91 ± 0.02	0.97 ± 0.01
	500	90.98 ± 1.43	0.82 ± 0.03	0.91 ± 0.02	0.91 ± 0.02	0.97 ± 0.01
SVM	Poly (Linear)	70.03 ± 1.93	0.40 ± 0.04	0.69 + 0.03	0.71 ± 0.03	0.70 ± 0.02
	Poli 2	78.41 ± 1.83	0.57 ± 0.04	0.78 ±0.03	0.79 ± 0.03	0.78 ± 0.02
	Poli 3	82.02 ± 1.77	0.64 ± 0.04	0.81 ± 0.03	0.83 ± 0.02	0.82 ± 0.02
SVM	RBF 0.1	70.05 ± 1.94	0.40 ± 0.04	0.70 ± 0.03	0.70 ± 0.03	0.70 ± 0.02
	RBF 0.2	73.47 ± 1.97	0.47 ± 0.04	0.75 ± 0.03	0.72 ± 0.03	0.73 ± 0.02
	RBF 0.5	78.30 ± 1.81	0.57 ± 0.04	0.79 ± 0.03	0.77 ± 0.03	0.78 ± 0.02

To simplify the problem, reduce dimensionality, and raise success rates, this study now explores other regions and methodologies. We estimate all missing signals to build a complete dataset and carry out further investigations.

4.2 Complete Base

Table 5 shows that Naive Bayes yields unsatisfactory results. It obtains the lowest metrics among all classifiers, with an accuracy of 58.58%, a Kappa Index of 0.17, a sensitivity of 0.25, and an AUC of 0.60. Its specificity of 0.92 stands as the only exception. These values suggest an almost random approach to detecting ASD. Bayes Net performs better, achieving 74.2% accuracy and a higher ability to identify true positives (sensitivity).

In this analysis, the tree-based models stand out with significantly superior performance. Both Decision Trees and Random Forest achieve accuracies, sensitivities, and specificities above 90%. Random Decision Tree, however, reports an 80% Kappa Index, which suggests lower agreement between training and validation. Random Forest with 100 and 500 trees produces exceptional outcomes, showing accuracies above 98% and near-ideal sensitivity and specificity for detecting ASD and identifying the control group.

SVMs deliver the best overall performance. Polynomial kernel models of degrees 1, 2, and 3 reach accuracies of 96%, 97%, and 98%, with true positive and true negative rates also near 98%. The SVM with an RBF kernel of degree 0.1 stands out the most. It attains a 99.13% accuracy and a 0.44 standard deviation, surpassing every other model. These findings reveal multiple opportunities to refine hyperparameters and further boost final performance.

We used GIMP Version 2.10.34 (Oliver et al., 2006) to compute the coordinates of all 64 electrodes. Equation 2 measures the distance between two electrodes, where "*a*" and "*b*" indicate the points, and "*x*1"/"*y*1" and "*x*2"/"*y*2" refer to their respective coordinates. After the interpolation process, GNU Octave 8.2.0 (Eaton et al., 2023) segmented the data into windows and extracted relevant attributes. Each window yielded 34 attributes, including mean, variance, standard deviation, root mean square, and mean amplitude variation. With 64 electrodes, we obtained 2,176 total attributes, which have proven relevance in earlier studies on EEG and peripheral physiological signals (de Santana et al., 2023). Each window spans 2 seconds, with a 0.5-second overlap and a 512 Hz sampling frequency. An Evolutionary Search method then selected the most significant attributes.

4.3 PSO

Table 6 displays the results of the training and validation phases after feature selection with PSO. These data reveal a wide performance gap among models.

Table 5 Results of the training and validation stage of the complete dataset, with all 64 electrodes and features. Approach 1.

Classifier		*Accuracy (%)*	*Kappa Index*	*Sensitivity*	*Specificity*	*AUC*
Bayes Net	-	74.20 ± 2.07	0.48 ± 0.04	0.76 ± 0.03	0.72 ± 0.03	0.81 ± 0.02
Naive Bayes	-	58.58 ± 1.67	0.17 ± 0.03	0.25 ± 0.03	0.92 ± 0.02	0.60 ± 0.02
Random Tree	-	90.04 ± 1.38	0.80 ± 0.03	0.90 ± 0.02	0.90 ± 0.02	0.90 ± 0.01
Rdm Forest	10	95.66 ± 0.99	0.91 ± 0.02	0.97 ± 0.01	0.94 ± 0.02	0.99 ± 0.00
	100	98.33 ± 0.59	0.97 ± 0.01	0.98 ± 0.01	0.98 ± 0.01	1.00 ± 0.00
	500	98.54 ± 0.54	0.91 ± 0.01	0.99 ± 0.01	0.98 ± 0.01	1.00 + 0.00
SVM	Poly (Linear)	96.36 ± 0.87	0.93 ± 0.02	0.96 ± 0.01	0.97 ± 0.01	0.96 ± 0.01
	Poli 2	97.84 ± 0.69	0.96 ± 0.01	0.98 ±0.01	0.98 ± 0.01	0.98 ± 0.01
	Poli 3	98.15 ± 0.79	0.96 ± 0.02	0.98 ± 0.01	0.98 ± 0.01	0.98 ± 0.01
SVM	RBF 0.5	92.99 ± 1.50	0.86 ± 0.03	0.98 ± 0.01	0.88 ± 0.03	0.93 ± 0.01
	RBF 0.2	98.24 ± 0.59	0.96 ± 0.01	0.99 ± 0.01	0.97 ± 0.01	0.98 ± 0.01
	RBF 0.1	**99.13 ± 0.44**	**0.98 ± 0.01**	**0.99 ± 0.01**	**0.99 ± 0.01**	**0.99 ± 0.00**

Table 6 Results of the training and validation phase of the dataset after PSO. Approach 2.

Classifier		*Accuracy (%)*	*Kappa Index*	*Sensitivity*	*Specificity*	*AUC*
Bayes Net	-	74.26 ± 2.09	0.49 ± 0.04	0.80 ± 0.03	0.69 ± 0.03	0.82 ± 0.02
Naive Bayes	-	59.44 ± 1.59	0.19 ± 0.03	0.27 ± 0.03	0.91 ± 0.02	0.75 ± 0.02
Random Tree	-	90.55 ± 1.49	0.81 ± 0.03	0.91 ± 0.02	0.90 ± 0.02	0.91 ± 0.01
Random Forest	10	95.87 ± 0.94	0.92 ± 0.02	0.98 ± 0.01	0.94 ± 0.02	0.99 ± 0.00
	100	98.21 ± 0.61	0.96 ± 0.01	0.98 ± 0.01	0.98 ± 0.01	1.00 ± 0.00
	500	98.37 ± 0.57	0.97 ± 0.01	0.99 ± 0.01	0.98 ± 0.01	1.00 ± 0.00
SVM	Poly (Linear)	92.33 ± 1.11	0.84 ± 0.02	0.91 ± 0.01	0.92 ± 0.01	0.92 ± 0.01
	Poli 2	98.17 ± 0.58	0.96 ± 0.01	0.98 ± 0.00	0.98 ± 0.00	0.98 ± 0.00
	Poli 3	98.48 ± 0.53	0.96 ± 0.01	0.98 ± 0.00	0.98 ± 0.00	0.98 ± 0.00
SVM	RBF 0.5	98.86 ± 0.51	0.97 ± 0.01	0.99 ± 0.00	0.98 ± 0.00	0.98 ± 0.01
	RBF 0.2	**99.23 ± 0.38**	**0.98 ± 0.00**	**0.99 ± 0.00**	**0.99 ± 0.00**	**0.99 ± 0.00**
	RBF 0.1	98.50 ± 0.55	0.97 ± 0.01	0.98 ± 0.00	0.98 ± 0.00	0.98 ± 0.00

The difference between the average accuracies of the best and worst models reaches 39.74%. This finding underscores the importance of choosing the right features for effective classification.

Table 2 shows that PSO significantly reduces the database size. The number of attributes drops from 2,142 (34 for each of the 63 electrodes) to 686. This reduction speeds up processing and preserves the classifiers' effectiveness, which remains solid and comparable to the previous approach.

Among simpler algorithms, Naive Bayes remains the weakest performer during training. It shows a small improvement in key metrics compared to the previous approach, but sensitivity in ASD classification still poses its main challenge. Bayes Net and Random Tree continue as the second and third worst models.

The SVM with RBF kernel and gamma 0.2 reaches remarkable results, including 99.23% accuracy, a 0.98 Kappa Index, 0.99 sensitivity, 0.99 specificity, and a 0.99 AUC. Despite the significant drop in the number of attributes, these metrics stay near 100%. Other SVM configurations, except for the one with a linear polynomial kernel, post results close to the top model.

Random Forest configurations, both the simpler version with 10 trees and the extended version with 500 trees, surpass 90% in all metrics. Their lower computational cost makes them a practical alternative.

4.4 9 (Nine) Electrodes

Table 7 shows the results obtained by using 9 manually selected electrodes. The difference between the best and worst model reaches 37 percentage points. Naive Bayes performs the worst, with an accuracy of 61%, a Kappa Index of 0.20, and a sensitivity of 26%, aligning with its weak performance in the other approaches. Bayes Net performs better than Naive Bayes, reaching 73.26% accuracy.

Among the tree-based models, Random Tree reached 89.91% accuracy, with sensitivity, specificity, and area under the ROC curve at 90%. These metrics indicate strong classification of both positives and negatives. However, Random Forest surpassed Random Tree regardless of the number of trees (10, 100, or 500). Its performance remained consistent, and the configuration with 500 trees recorded 98% accuracy. It also had sensitivity and specificity higher than 98%, which are essential indicators for differentiating ASD and the control group.

Even with fewer electrodes, the results stayed impressive. Using all 34 attributes for each of the 9 selected electrodes appeared more effective than using fewer attributes spread across more channels, as seen in the evolutionary search. SVMs had performance slightly below that of Random Forest. The

Table 7 Results of the training and validation stage of the dataset after manual selection of 9 electrodes of the frontotemporal group. Approach 3.

Classifier		*Accuracy (%)*	*Kappa Index*	*Sensitivity*	*Specificity*	*AUC*
Bayes Net	-	73.26 ± 2.09	0.47 ± 0.04	0.75 ± 0.03	0.72 ± 0.03	0.83 ± 0.02
Naive Bayes	-	61.01 ± 0.65	0.20 ± 0.03	0.26 ± 0.02	0.93 ± 0.01	0.74 ± 0.02
Random Tree	-	89.91 ± 1.70	0.80 ± 0.03	0.90 ± 0.02	0.90 ± 0.02	0.90 ± 0.02
Rdm Forest	10	96.14 ± 0.94	0.92 ± 0.02	0.98 ± 0.01	0.95 ± 0.02	0.99 ± 0.00
	100	97.91 ± 0.68	0.96 ± 0.01	0.98 ± 0.01	0.97 ± 0.01	1.00 ± 0.00
	500	**98.06 ± 0.66**	**0.96 ± 0.01**	**0.99 ± 0.01**	**0.98 ± 0.01**	**1.00 ± 0.00**
SVM	Poly (Linear)	84.48 ± 1.60	0.69 ± 0.03	0.84 ± 0.02	0.85 ± 0.02	0.84 ± 0.02
	Poli 2	96.39 ± 0.85	0.93 ± 0.02	0.96 ± 0.01	0.96 ± 0.01	0.96 ± 0.01
	Poli 3	96.57 ± 0.88	0.93 ± 0.02	0.96 ± 0.01	0.97 ± 0.01	0.97 ± 0.01
SVM	RBF 0.5	96.71 ± 0.80	0.93 ± 0.02	0.96 ± 0.01	0.97 ± 0.01	0.97 ± 0.01
	RBF 0.2	93.81 ± 1.10	0.88 ± 0.02	0.92 ± 0.02	0.95 ± 0.01	0.94 ± 0.01
	RBF 0.1	89.26 ± 1.37	0.79 ± 0.03	0.86 ± 0.02	0.93 ± 0.02	0.89 ± 0.01

SVM with a linear polynomial kernel was least effective, with 84.48% accuracy, 84% sensitivity, 85% specificity, and a 69% Kappa Index. The SVM with an RBF kernel and gamma of 0.5 achieved the highest accuracy at 96.71% (± 0.80). This figure was on par with the degree 2 and 3 polynomial SVMs, all within the same margin of error.

4.5 Testing the Best Models

We tested the top models of each approach (full dataset, PSO, and 9 electrodes) on independent samples in a single run. Table 8 presents the detailed results.

Table 8 Results of the test stage performed in a single round with the best models of each approach.

Classifier	*Accuracy (%)*	*Kappa Index*	*Sensitivity*	*Specificity*	*AUC*
64 electrodes SVM RBF 0.1	94.77	0.89	0.95	0.94	0.95
PSO SVM RBF 0.2	96.71	0.93	0.97	0.97	0.97
9 electrodes Random Forest 500	**99.74**	**0.99**	**0.99**	**0.99**	**1**

During the test, the three models performed well and yielded similar results. However, the SVM models for the complete dataset and after PSO showed slightly lower values for all five metrics. In this single round, the Random Forest model with manually selected electrodes delivered the best performance. It approached 100% accuracy and excelled in the other metrics. This outcome confirms the potential of these classifiers when confronted with new data.

We generated confusion matrices for each model, as shown in Figure 8. They offer a clearer view of true positives, true negatives, false positives, and false negatives predicted by each classifier.

(a)

	Classified ASD	Classified C
ASD	562	28
Control	34	561

(b)

	Classified ASD	Classified C
ASD	570	19
Control	20	576

(c)

	Classified ASD	Classified C
ASD	590	1
Control	2	591

Fig. 8 Confusion matrix of the test performed with (a) complete dataset and SVM model. (b) PSO and SVM model. (c) Manual selection of electrodes and Random Forest with 500 trees.

From Figure 8(a), we observe the SVM matrix with the complete dataset, which accurately classifies 562 windows from individuals in the ASD group and 561 windows from individuals in the control group. This balanced outcome aligns with the high sensitivity and specificity scores. Figure 8(b) shows similar rates for the SVM model tested on the PSO dataset. This model correctly classifies 570 ASD windows and 576 control windows. Finally, the model with 9 manually selected electrodes shows the best results, even though the testing was performed only once. It correctly classifies 590 ASD windows and 591 control windows. This success underscores the significance of this brain region for diagnosing ASD.

5. Conclusion

This chapter's primary goal was to develop an innovative method that supports the differential diagnosis of ASD by automatically analyzing low-density EEG signals. We employ advanced machine learning techniques to detect specific EEG patterns that characterize ASD. This framework has strong potential for enhancing diagnostic accuracy and speed, serving as a valuable complement to traditional methods.

Reflecting on the initial scope, the results are encouraging. Researchers have identified EEG patterns linked to ASD with notable accuracy. This milestone advances the field of diagnostics by reducing the time to diagnosis and enabling earlier, more personalized interventions for individuals with ASD. Moreover, introducing machine learning in this domain broadens research possibilities and fosters the development of more effective, accessible health technologies.

In this work, we used a public database containing EEG signals from autistic individuals of various ages. We first introduced an interpolation method to handle missing data, then applied particle swarm optimization and evolutionary search to select the most significant attributes. Bayesian models, decision trees, random forests, and SVMs emerged as classifiers during data analysis, achieving remarkably high-performance scores.

The methodology presented in this chapter has several notable strengths.

First, advanced machine learning methods and a careful selection of relevant features enabled us to detect discriminative EEG patterns linked to ASD. The interpolation method for missing signals significantly reduced data gaps. Researchers then chose to lower the number of electrodes and focus on a specific cortical region after reviewing studies that report distinct activation in those areas among ASD individuals. This strategy produced the best outcomes and simplified diagnostic support, making it more accessible and promoting early interventions. It also enhanced results for people with autism.

We must also recognize certain limitations. Variations in EEG acquisition protocols affected data consistency and comparability. The scarcity of public databases associating EEG with ASD posed another challenge. Additional validation in independent samples is vital to confirm the robustness and generalizability of the findings. Participant data only included age and class membership, which narrows the research scope. We also lack details about individual ASD levels. Researchers must consider these factors to support accurate interpretation and guide future studies toward more reliable outcomes.

Despite these constraints, this work offers essential contributions to public health. Comparative analysis: More efficient and accessible methods for diagnosing ASD can broaden access to early interventions and improve outcomes for individuals with the disorder. Automating diagnostic processes also reduces the time and costs usually involved in identifying ASD, a benefit for both patients and healthcare systems.

Acknowledgment(s)

We acknowledge partial financial support from the Brazilian research agencies National Council for Scientific and Technological Development (CNPq 304636/2021-5), Pernambuco State Science and Technology Support Foundation (FACEPE IBPG-2267-3.13/22), Coordination for the Improvement of Higher Education Personnel (CAPES), and the Studies and Projects Financing Agency (FINEP 2170/22).

Disclosure Statement

The authors declare no financial or non-financial conflicts of interest.

References

American Psychiatric Association. (2013). Diagnostic and statistical manual of mental disorders (5th Edn.). *American Psychiatric Association.*

Antunes, M.P., Rosa, J.L.G., Sabai, F.J. and de Aguiar Neto, F.S. (2023). Early detection of autism spectrum disorder using non-invasive EEG In: 2023 *IEEE 19th International Conference on Body Sensor Networks* (*BSN*), pp. 1–4. IEEE.

Atienza, D., Larrañaga, P. and Bielza, C. (2022). Hybrid semiparametric Bayesian networks. *TEST, 31*(2), 299–327.

Calomino, C., Bianco, M.G., Oliva, G., Laganà, F., Pullano, S.A. and Quattrone, A. 2024. Comparative analysis of cross-validation methods on PPMI dataset. In: *2024 IEEE International Symposium on Medical Measurements and Applications* (MeMeA), pp. 1–5. IEEE.

Cañete-Sifuentes, L., Monroy, R. and Medina-Pérez, M.A. (2021). A review and experimental comparison of multivariate decision trees. *IEEE Access, 9*, 110451–110479.

Chamasemani, F.F. and Singh, Y.P. (2011). Multi-class support vector machine (SVM) classifiers – An application in hypothyroid detection and classification. In: *2011 Sixth International Conference on Bio-Inspired Computing: Theories and Applications*, pp. 351–356. IEEE.

Chen, F.W. and Liu, C.W. (2012). Estimation of the spatial rainfall distribution using inverse distance weighting (IDW) in the middle of Taiwan. *Paddy and Water Environment, 10*, 209–222.

Chen, J., Wang, X. and Lei, F. (2024). Data-driven multinomial random forest: A new random forest variant with strong consistency. *Journal of Big Data, 11*(1), 34.

Darwiche, A. (2008). Bayesian networks. *Foundations of Artificial Intelligence*, *3*, 467–509.

de Almeida, W.F., de Moraes Lima, C.A. and Peres, S.M. (2021). A systematic mapping of feature extraction and feature selection methods of electroencephalogram signals for neurological diseases diagnostic assistance. *IEEE Latin America Transactions, 19*, 735–745.

de Menezes, J.A.A., Gomes, J.C., de Carvalho Hazin, V., Dantas, J.C.S., Rodrigues, M.C.A. and Dos Santos, W.P. (2023). Motor imagery classification using sparse representations: An exploratory study. *Scientific Reports*, *13*(1), 15585.

de Santana, M.A., Fonseca, F.S., Torcate, A.S. and dos Santos, W.P. (2023). Emotion recognition from multimodal data: A machine learning approach combining classical and hybrid deep architectures. *Research on Biomedical Engineering*, *39*, 613–639.

Delorme, A. and Makeig, S. (2004). EEGLAB: An open source toolbox for analysis of single-trial EEG dynamics including independent component analysis. *Journal of Neuroscience Methods*, *134*(1), 9–21.

Dickinson, A., Jeste, S. and Milne, E. (2022). Electrophysiological signatures of brain aging in autism spectrum disorder. *Cortex*, *148*, 139–151.

Dimitoglou, G., Adams, J.A. and Jim, C.M. (2012). Comparison of the C4.5 and a naïve Bayes classifier for the prediction of lung cancer survivability. *arXiv Preprint*. https://arxiv.org/abs/1206.1121.

Dong, L., Du, H., Mao, F., Han, N., Li, X., Zhou, G., Zheng, J., Zhang, M., Xing, L., Liu, T., et al. (2019). Very high resolution remote sensing imagery classification using a fusion of random forest and deep learning technique: Subtropical area, for example. *IEEE Journal of Selected Topics in Applied Earth Observations and Remote Sensing, 13*, 113–128.

Duan, L., Duan, H., Qiao, Y., Sha, S., Qi, S., Zhang, X., Huang, J., Huang, X. and Wang, C. (2020). Machine learning approaches for MDD detection and emotion decoding using EEG signals. *Frontiers in Human Neuroscience, 14*. https://doi.org/10.3389/fnhum.2020.00009.

Eaton, J.W., Bateman, D., Hauberg, S. and Wehbring, R. (2023). *GNU Octave Version 8.4.0 Manual: A High-level Interactive Language for Numerical Computations.* https://octave.org/doc/v8.4.0/.

Eibe, F., Hall, M.A., Witten, I.H. and Pal, J. (2016). *The Weka Workbench. Online Appendix for Data Mining: Practical Machine Learning Tools and Techniques* (4th Edn.).

Fonseca, F.S., Torcate, A.S., Da Silva, A.C.G., Freire, V.H.W., De Farias, G.P.D.M., De Oliveira, J.F.L., De Oliveira Júnior, F.M.D., De Souza Júnior, J.C.D.S., Gomes, D.A. and Dos Santos, W.P. (2022). Early prediction of generalized infection in intensive care units from clinical data: A committee-based machine learning approach. In: 2022 *IEEE Latin American Conference on Computational Intelligence* (*LA-CCI*), pp. 1–6. IEEE.

Gomes, J.C., de Freitas Barbosa, V.A., de Santana, M.A., de Lima, C.L., Calado, R.B., Barbosa Júnior, C.R., de Almeida Albuquerque, J.E., de Souza, R.G., de Araújo, R.J.E., Moreno, G.M.M., et al. (2023). Rapid protocols to support COVID-19 clinical diagnosis based on hematological parameters. *Research on Biomedical Engineering, 39*(3), 509–539.

Hall, M., Frank, E., Holmes, G., Pfahringer, B., Reutemann, P. and Witten, I.H. (2009). The WEKA data mining software: An update. *ACM SIGKDD Explorations Newsletter, 11*(1), 10–18.

Hao, C., Chen, C., Wen, Y., Meng, F., Chi, Z., Zhao, R., Wu, Y., Lian, Q., Wang, L., Li, P. and Cheng, L. (2023). Research progress of electroencephalogram (EEG) classification method and its application based on support vector machine (SVM). In: *2023 16th International Congress on Image and Signal Processing, BioMedical Engineering and Informatics* (CISP-BMEI), pp. 1–4. IEEE.

Heinsfeld, A.S., Franco, A.R., Craddock, R.C., Buchweitz, A. and Meneguzzi, F. (2018). Identification of autism spectrum disorder using deep learning and the ABIDE dataset. *NeuroImage: Clinical, 17*, 16–23.

Kemp, B. and Olivan, J. (2003). European data format 'plus' (EDF+), an EDF alike standard format for the exchange of physiological data. *Clinical Neurophysiology, 114*(9), 1755–1761.

Khodatars, M., Shoeibi, A., Sadeghi, D., Ghaasemi, N., Jafari, M., Moridian, P., Khadem, A., Alizadehsani, R., Zare, A., Kong, Y., et al. (2021). Deep learning for neuroimaging-based diagnosis and rehabilitation of autism spectrum disorder: A review. *Computers in Biology and Medicine, 139*, 104949.

Kim, T. and Lee, J.-S. (2022). Exponential loss minimization for learning weighted naive Bayes classifiers. *IEEE Access, 10*, 22724–22736.

Kong, X., Li, J. and Ouyang, G. (2023). EEG microstate analysis for diagnosis of children with ASD. In: *2023 42nd Chinese Control Conference* (*CCC*), pp. 3390–3395. IEEE.

Kulage, K.M., Smaldone, A.M. and Cohn, E.G. (2014). How will DSM-5 affect autism diagnosis? A systematic literature review and meta-analysis. *Journal of Autism and Developmental Disorders, 44*, 1918–1932.

Kulage, K.M., Goldberg, J., Usseglio, J., Romero, D., Bain, J.M. and Smaldone, A.M. (2020). How has DSM-5 affected autism diagnosis? A 5-year follow-up systematic literature review and meta-analysis. *Journal of Autism and Developmental Disorders, 50*, 2102–2127.

Kumar, R., Bordoloi, D., Shrivastava, A., Kumar, C.P., Kumari, V. and Kumar, A. (2023). Behavioral and clinical data analysis for autism spectrum disorder screening with machine learning. In: *2023 10th IEEE Uttar Pradesh Section International Conference on Electrical, Electronics, and Computer Engineering* (*UPCON*) (Vol. 10), pp. 1803–1810. IEEE.

Li, B., Cheng, T. and Guo, Z. (2021). A review of EEG acquisition, processing, and application. In: *Journal of Physics: Conference Series* (Vol. 1907), p. 012045. IOP Publishing.

Li, Z. and Wang, P. (2013). Intelligent optimization on power values for inverse distance weighting. In: *2013 International Conference on Information Science and Cloud Computing Companion*, pp. 370–375. IEEE.

Lord, C., Elsabbagh, M., Baird, G. and Veenstra-Vanderweele, J. (2018). Autism spectrum disorder. *The Lancet, 392*(10146), 508–520.

Lord, C., Brugha, T.S., Charman, T., Cusack, J., Dumas, G., Frazier, T., Jones, E.J., Jones, R.M. and Pickles, A. (2020). Autism spectrum disorder. *Nature Reviews Disease Primers, 6*(5).

Mahadevkar, S.V., Khemani, B., Patil, S., Kotecha, K., Vora, D.R., Abraham, A. and Gabralla, L.A. (2022). A review on machine learning styles in computer vision: Techniques and future directions. *IEEE Access, 10*, 107293–107329.

Malmivuo, J. and Plonsey, R. (1995). Bioelectromagnetism: principles and applications of bioelectric and biomagnetic fields. Oxford university press.

Niranjan, A., Nutan, D., Nitish, A., Deepa-Shenoy, P., Venugopal, K. and ERCR, T. (2018). Ensemble of random committee and random tree for efficient anomaly classification using voting. In: *Proceedings of the International Conference for Convergence in Technology,* Pune, India, pp. 6–8. IEEE.

Nunes, I.B., de Santana, M.A., Charron, N., de. Silva, H.S., de Lima Simões, C.M., Lins, C., de Souza Sampaio, A.B., de Melo, A.M.N., da Silva, T.C.V., Tiodista, C., et al. (2024). Automatic identification of preferred music genres: An exploratory machine learning approach to support personalized music therapy. *Multimedia Tools and Applications*, 1–17.

Oktavia, E., Widyawan and Mustika, I.W. (2016). Inverse distance weighting and kriging spatial interpolation for data center thermal monitoring. In: *2016 1st International Conference on Information Technology, Information Systems, and Electrical Engineering* (*ICITISEE*), pp. 69–74. IEEE.

Oliver, E., Ruiz, J., She, S. and Wang, J. (2006). The software architecture of the GIMP. *Retrieved from [original publication details missing].*

Oostenveld, R. and Praamstra, P. (2001). The five percent electrode system for high-resolution EEG and ERP measurements. *Clinical Neurophysiology*, *112*(4), 713–719.

Pagnozzi, A.M., Conti, E., Calderoni, S., Fripp, J. and Rose, S.E. (2018). A systematic review of structural MRI biomarkers in autism spectrum disorder: A machine learning perspective. *International Journal of Developmental Neuroscience, 71*, 68–82.

Patil, S. and Patil, P. (2023). A clinical diagnosis-based approach for EEG-based classification of autism spectrum disorder using Hilbert transform and single label SVM. In: *2023 7th International Conference On Computing, Communication, Control, and Automation* (*ICCUBEA*), pp. 1–6. IEEE.

P.D., W.M. and Haryoko. (2022). Improved support vector machine (SVM) performance on Go-Jek service review classification using particle swarm optimization (PSO). In: *2022 International Conference on Informatics, Multimedia, Cyber, and Information System* (*ICIMCIS*), pp. 298–301. IEEE. doi: 10.1109/ICIMCIS56303.2022.10017911.

Rani, A., Yadav, P. and Verma, Y. (2022). Early-stage autism diagnosis using action videos and contrastive feature learning. *Multimedia Systems, 29*, 2603–2614.

Saleem, K., Khan, M.S.G., Firdous, A., Naseer, I., Rashid, A., Saleem, S. and Naseer, A. (2021). Diagnostic evaluation of autism spectrum disorders, a health professional survey. *Journal of Pharmaceutical Research International.*

Sari, Y., Baskara, A.R. and Wahyuni, R. (2021). Classification of chili leaf disease using the gray level co-occurrence matrix (GLCM) and the support vector machine (SVM) methods. In: *2021 Sixth International Conference on Informatics and Computing (ICIC)*, pp. 1–4. IEEE.

Shubho, S.A., Razib, M.R.H., Rudro, N.K., Saha, A.K., Khan, M.S.U. and Ahmed, S. (2019). Performance analysis of NB Tree, REP Tree, and Random Tree classifiers for credit card fraud data. In: *2019 22nd International Conference on Computer and Information Technology (ICCIT)*, pp. 1–6. IEEE.

Tarca, A.L., Carey, V.J., Chen, X.-W., Romero, R. and Draghici, S. (2007). Machine learning and its applications to biology. *PLoS Computational Biology*, *3*(6), e116.

Van Rossum, G. and Drake, F.L. (2009). *Python 3 Reference Manual.* CreateSpace.

Vandekar, S.N., Shinohara, R.T., Raznahan, A., Roalf, D.R., Ross, M., DeLeo, N., Ruparel, K., Verma, R., Wolf, D.H., Gur, R.C., et al. (2015). Topologically dissociable patterns of development of the human cerebral cortex. *Journal of Neuroscience, 35*(2), 599–609.

Volkmar, F.R. and Reichow, B. (2013). Autism in DSM-5: Progress and challenges. *Molecular Autism*, *4*, 1–6.

Wu, X., Liu, H., Zhang, L., Skibniewski, M.J., Deng, Q. and Teng, J. (2015). A dynamic Bayesian network based approach to safety decision support in tunnel construction. *Reliability Engineering and System Safety, 134*, 157–168.

Yoo, H. (2016). Early detection and intervention of autism spectrum disorder. *Hanyang Medical Reviews, 36*, 4–10.

Yuan, D., Huang, J., Yang, X. and Cui, J. (2020). Improved random forest classification approach based on hybrid clustering selection. In: *2020 Chinese Automation Congress (CAC)*, (pp. 1559–1563). IEEE.

Zhao, P., Zhang, L., Liu, G. and Si, S. (2011). Design and development of the Bayesian network platform based on B/S structure. In: *2011 Fourth International Symposium on Knowledge Acquisition and Modeling*, pp. 65–68. IEEE.

8 | Innovations and Emerging Technologies in the Context of Autism Spectrum Disorders (ASD)

Carlo Marcelo Revoredo da Silva[1*] and Vanderlene Covre Rocha[1,2]

This chapter presents a comprehensive overview of innovations and emerging technologies for assessing and supporting individuals with Autism Spectrum Disorder (ASD). It begins by outlining the evolution of diagnostic criteria and highlighting the importance of early detection to improve interventions and family support. Traditional methods are critiqued, emphasizing the need for rigorous, evidence-based practices that address sociocultural biases and diverse presentations. Artificial Intelligence (AI) then emerges as a valuable tool, offering enhanced diagnostic precision, efficiency, and scalability through machine learning, deep learning, and generative models. The text also explores the use of Virtual and Augmented Reality, wearable sensors, and games to create immersive, personalized, and inclusive approaches. Biomedical Engineering contributions include imaging techniques (EEG, fMRI, MRI) and signal processing to refine diagnostics and guide targeted therapies. Finally, the chapter discusses integrative strategies that unite AI, Neuroscience, and Engineering, while reflecting on ethical implications, privacy safeguards, and transparent decision-making.

1. Introduction to Autism Spectrum Disorders (ASD)

Over the last few decades, perspectives on Autism Spectrum Disorder (ASD) changed in a significant way. Scientific advances and shifts in diagnostic criteria guided this evolution. Public policies and educational practices also matured during this period. This transformation refined our understanding of ASD. It encouraged more effective, innovative, and humanized interventions. Knowledge of the historical path and the various factors in the spectrum supports more conscious inclusion. It ensures adequate family support. It improves the quality of life for individuals within this broad and diverse setting.

[1] Universidade de Pernambuco, Pernambuco, Brazil.
[2] Instituto Federal do Pará, Pará, Brazil.
* Corresponding author: cmrs@poli.br.

DOI: 10.1201/9781003531418-8

1.1 The Concept of Autism Over Time

Scientists and society changed the view on autism significantly since the first clinical descriptions in the early 20th century. In the 1940s, psychiatrist Leo Kanner described for the first time a group of children with marked difficulties in social interaction, communication, and restricted and repetitive behaviors. He created the term "early infantile autism" (Kanner, 1943). At the same time, Austrian physician Hans Asperger acted independently. He identified similar traits in children who had social difficulties but also preserved or advanced linguistic skills in certain domains. His descriptions led to the concept of "Asperger Syndrome" (Asperger, 1991).

In subsequent decades, professionals no longer viewed autism as a rare, rigid condition. They placed it in a broader spectrum of clinical presentations. Researchers refined diagnostic criteria. They used new findings and professional expertise. Cultural, social, and scientific factors influenced the expansion and revision of the definition of autism. The *DSM-5*[1] (Association, 2013, 2022) officially adopted the term ASD instead of separate diagnostic entities. This new perspective recognizes that autism's characteristics vary greatly in intensity and form of expression. It creates a more inclusive and dynamic view of the condition.

1.2 Brief Overview of ASD

ASD, as defined today, includes a wide range of conditions with difficulties in social interaction, communication, and restricted or repetitive behaviors, interests, and activities (Silva and Mulick, 2009). This variety of manifestations creates a heterogeneous condition. Some individuals show marked impairments in speech and social understanding. Others display specific cognitive abilities or talents in limited areas. The spectrum includes nonverbal people or those with intellectual difficulties. It also includes those with typical or even above-average cognitive abilities, who still face challenges in subtle areas of social communication and behavior (Tsai, et al., 2020).

1.3 Importance of Early Detection

Early detection of ASD signs stands as a critical factor for effective interventions and child development. The sooner professionals confirm the diagnosis, the sooner they can introduce individualized therapies that support communication, social interaction, and adaptation to the environment (Bradshaw, et al., 2020; Fuller and Kaiser, 2020). This identification can

---

[1] https://www.psychiatry.org/psychiatrists/practice/dsm.

occur in the first years of life. Signs may include inadequate eye contact, lack of response when called by name, restricted interests, and delays in speech development.

Early diagnosis also benefits families. They gain guidance and support in understanding challenges, setting routines, and promoting essential skills in the child (Zwaigenbaum, et al., 2021). Early involvement of specialized professionals helps schools and other social environments prepare to welcome and assist children. This approach encourages inclusion. Investment in early detection and intervention fosters better outcomes in development, learning, and social integration.

Furthermore, inclusive education creates significant challenges for teachers and school managers. They must adapt curricula, pedagogical strategies, and teaching materials to address cognitive and behavioral diversity (Caputo, Iervese, and Isidori, 2020). Specialized Educational Assistance (SEA) complements the standard education of students with special educational needs. It includes activities, resources, accessibility measures, and pedagogical strategies. These elements provide more appropriate support for atypical students (Lima and Angelo, 2024; Luz et al., 2024).

Active family involvement and clinical guidance are essential. Specialists gather assessments and evidence-based data on each student's characteristics and needs. This information guides pedagogues and educators in forming individualized plans (Costa, Schmidt, and Camargo, 2023), such as the Individualized Educational Plan (IEP) and the Individual Development Plan (IDP). This approach fosters a supportive, responsive, and effective learning environment for both academic and social development.

2. Current Diagnostic Scenario

Health professionals currently rely on increasingly comprehensive criteria to diagnose ASD. These criteria reflect the multiple and complex variations in its clinical presentations. Advancements in neuroscience, genetics, and developmental psychology have introduced more sophisticated and multidisciplinary diagnostic tools. These tools consider not only classic behavioral indicators but also neurobiological and environmental factors. However, the spectrum's heterogeneity and the need for early, accurate diagnoses pose continuous challenges. Professionals now rethink how they assess and identify ASD. They seek more efficient, sensitive, and culturally appropriate approaches. This scenario combines an expanded base of scientific knowledge with an urgent call to turn these insights into more inclusive and effective diagnostic strategies.

2.1 Physiology of ASD

Experts see ASD as the result of a complex interaction among genetic, epigenetic, environmental, and neurodevelopmental factors (Chahin, et al., 2020). Neuroimaging studies show changes in the connectivity and structure of certain brain regions, especially those linked to communication, social perception, and sensory regulation. In parallel, genetic and epigenetic research points to the influence of multiple genes, as well as the prenatal environment, in shaping ASD risk (Rolland, et al., 2019). Researchers also investigate the immunological and metabolic aspects of this condition.

No single or definitive biological marker exists at present. Still, converging findings from neuroimaging, genetic, biochemical, and systemic physiology suggest a highly complex neurobiological phenomenon. This perspective creates pathways for specific, personalized interventions that address the many dimensions of the spectrum.

2.2 Criticism of Traditional Methods

Traditional diagnostic methods rely heavily on brief clinical observations and parental reports. Specialists highlight serious flaws in these approaches. Cultural, gender, or social biases may affect results. Professionals often use behavioral scales and semi-structured interviews. These tools may not capture the full complexity and diversity of the spectrum, especially in different sociocultural contexts. They also demand significant time and resources. Families in vulnerable situations often lack access. This reality increases inequalities. It creates a cycle where only a small group receives accurate diagnoses and effective interventions.

Before we explore diagnostic challenges and new possibilities with Artificial Intelligence (AI), we note the inherent flaws in traditional methods. Many ASD diagnoses still arise from one or a few clinical evaluation sessions. Sometimes, a single consultation of about one hour decides the outcome. This practice raises questions about reliability and consistency. Multiple variables exist, such as the individual's emotional state and the clinician's subjectivity (Bauman 2010; Dauchez, et al., 2022; Defresne and Mottron, 2022). This limited model contrasts with the continuous and dynamic nature of human development. It obstructs a thorough understanding of the individual's needs and characteristics over time.

When we reflect on these limitations, we must consider the debate about the uncritical use of instruments and practices that lack scientific validation (Lacerda, 2023). In the ASD context, as in special education, we must rely on methods grounded in solid evidence and scientific rigor. We must avoid unproven or dubious strategies. This approach includes the adoption of new technologies, such as eye tracking systems, genetic marker analysis, and deep learning neural networks. Researchers, clinicians, families, and the person on the spectrum must evaluate these innovations carefully. By prioritizing evidence-based approaches and the active involvement of all stakeholders, we move toward more inclusive, precise, and fair diagnoses. This strategy reduces the risks of pseudoscience and supports the genuine well-being of people with ASD.

2.3 Existing Challenges

ASD diagnosis still poses major difficulties, despite more advanced diagnostic guidelines and protocols. One key barrier lies in the variability of clinical presentations. Some individuals show global developmental delays or communicative limitations. Others reveal only subtle behavior or interest patterns. The shortage of qualified professionals and the limited availability of specialized centers also hamper comprehensive assessments.

No single biological marker exists for ASD (Gupta and State, 2006; Taveira, et al., 2023). Professionals depend mostly on behavioral observations and family reports. This approach may lead to under- or overdiagnosis, plus delays in detection and early interventions. Socio cultural factors, such as prejudice, stigma, and a lack of awareness, further increase the complexity of diagnosis.

In this context, the use of AI for predicting and identifying ASD faces additional obstacles. The spectrum's extreme heterogeneity makes it difficult for predictive models to recognize consistent patterns in individuals with very different clinical and social profiles. The absence of biological markers and reliance on unstructured behavioral data also complicate algorithm development and can introduce biases (Song, et al., 2019).

Strategies that combine data from genomic, physiological, environmental, and behavioral sources help overcome these barriers. Diverse and representative databases also reinforce robustness in AI models (Joudar, et al., 2023; Wankhede, et al., 2024). Such methods reduce uncertainties, facilitate earlier and more accurate detection, and ensure fairer diagnoses.

3. Artificial Intelligence (AI) in Autism Detection

AI emerges as a promising strategy in mental health. It aims to improve the diagnosis and follow-up of complex conditions such as ASD (Lai, Lombardo, and Baron-Cohen, 2020). Algorithms learn from data. They identify subtle patterns and reveal statistical relationships across multiple variables. AI offers sensitive, objective, and scalable tools for clinical assessment. It surpasses human observation. It incorporates data from many sources, such as behavioral signals and gaze patterns (Wei, et al., 2023), executive functions (Townes, et al., 2023), and genetic data, physiological parameters, and medical histories (Brueggeman, Koomar, and Michaelson 2020). These data sets help create accurate predictive models that support the diagnostic process (Voss, Schafer, and Faja, 2021). AI can complement traditional methods. It adds precision, speed, and accessibility to ASD detection. This approach is especially vital in scenarios where specialists are scarce.

3.1 Machine Learning Approaches

Machine learning (ML) uses techniques that let computers identify patterns and make data-driven decisions, without explicit programming for each task (Russell and Norvig, 2021). In ASD contexts, specialists apply these approaches to analyze recordings of social interactions, examine difficulties in emotion recognition (alexithymia), detect facial expressions, assess voice intonation, or study body movement patterns. Sensing peripherals, discussed in Section 3.3, often support these tasks. Researchers use statistical algorithms and mathematical models to extract relevant features. They develop classifiers that distinguish individuals with and without ASD, often reaching accuracy rates similar to those of human experts.

ML can also include multimodal data analysis. It integrates information from various sensory sources and modalities—images, audio, and text—to create a more comprehensive diagnostic framework (Zhu, et al., 2023). Large, diverse datasets make these methods more scalable. They help reduce bias and improve generalization of results.

3.2 Deep Learning Models

Deep learning advances ML through artificial neural networks with multiple layers. These networks learn complex representations of data. They recognize subtle patterns and extract features without manual engineering. In ASD, researchers use convolutional neural networks (CNNs) to process images, videos, or biometric signals. They rely on recurrent neural networks (RNNs) to analyze sequences of behavior, speech, or text from clinical reports.

In recent years, the Transformers architecture revolutionized deep learning, especially in Natural Language Processing (NLP). This innovation led to major advances in Generative AI (GenAI) and Large Language Models (LLMs), such as GPT[2] and BERT[3]. They show remarkable effectiveness in complex

---

2 https://openai.com/chatgpt/overview/.

3 https://huggingface.co/docs/transformers/model doc/bert.

tasks of textual analysis, language generation, and semantic understanding (Vaswani, et al., 2023). In the context of ASD, these technologies broaden diagnostic and intervention possibilities. They enable the analysis of large volumes of multimodal data. They also personalize recommendations and support strategies, expanding solution accessibility.

Deep learning models handle large quantities of unstructured data. This ability holds special value for autism diagnosis, where signs appear in varied and nonlinear ways. For instance, neural networks can analyze children's social interaction videos. They identify facial microexpressions, eye contact patterns, and subtle hand gestures. The human eye often misses these details, though they serve as predictive markers for early diagnosis. As research progresses, deep learning will integrate further into assessment routines. This approach supports more individualized diagnoses.

With the rise of LLMs, new paths emerge for diagnosing and understanding ASD. These technologies assist in analyzing written clinical data, summarizing medical records, classifying symptom information, or suggesting diagnostic hypotheses. They also generate personalized scenarios and questions for interactive assessments. They simulate social or communicative situations. Their flexibility in natural language opens possibilities for large-scale screening tools, accessible to families and professionals in different sociocultural settings. By adding GenAI and LLMs to diagnostic processes, experts expect better accuracy, efficiency, and reach. This strategy fosters earlier diagnoses, more targeted interventions, and a notable improvement in support for people with ASD and their caregivers.

3.3 Emerging Technologies and Human-Computer Interfaces (HCI)

In addition to AI advances, several emerging technologies enhance detection, diagnosis, and intervention in ASD. Innovators integrate devices and interfaces such as Virtual Reality (VR), Augmented Reality (AR), Internet of Things (IoT), wearable devices, mobile devices, and games. These tools gather data in settings that resemble daily life, reduce biases, and produce more engaging and meaningful assessments. VR and AR create simulated and controlled scenarios that offer richer and more adaptable social, communicative, and sensory interactions than those found in a typical clinical office (Dechsling, et al., 2022). Glasses, headphones, and controllers monitor behavior, eye orientation (eye tracking), emotional responses, and reaction times (Asmetha Jeyarani and Senthilkumar 2023). This approach complements traditional strategies. It supplies professionals and researchers with details about behavioral patterns in environments close to real life, but under the security and control of a virtual setting.

IoT, combined with mobile devices and wearable sensors, gathers data beyond the lab or clinic. It records physiological, environmental, and behavioral indicators in real time during an individual's routine (Ghosh, et al., 2021). Devices like wristbands, smartwatches, headbands, and motion sensors offer continuous information about sleep patterns, physical activity, sensory reactivity, and social interactions. This knowledge fosters a deeper understanding of the person's ASD profile. It also supports personalized and adaptive interventions.

Peripherals such as microphones and speakers play key roles in collecting and presenting real-time information with the help of AI algorithms. Microphones and speech recognition systems convert speech to text, generating detailed and structured data for analyzing linguistic patterns, intonation, and other verbal nuances (Cassidy, et al., 2016). Speakers with speech synthesis tools convey instructions, feedback, and auditory stimuli clearly, keeping users engaged (Lee, et al., 2024). By transcribing human speech and delivering auditory communication, these peripherals broaden data collection options and improve user experiences. They serve as valuable resources for building responsive, inclusive, and informative environments.

Finally, games that match the individual's needs create playful and appealing experiences. They foster active user participation. They also collect valuable data (Carneiro, et al., 2024). These games offer an interactive and motivating environment. They serve for both assessment and skill training in cognitive, socio-emotional, and communicative domains. They also track the individual's progress over time. Emerging technologies and HCI (human-computer interaction) interfaces, combined with AI solutions, form a promising ecosystem that improves data collection, reduces bias, and provides more inclusive and effective opportunities for supporting individuals with ASD.

4. Contributions of Biomedical Engineering

Biomedical Engineering plays an increasingly essential role in the identification, monitoring, and comprehension of ASD. It unites expertise from engineering, biology, information technology, and medicine. This field delivers new tools and approaches that surpass traditional clinical methods (Patel, et al., 2021). Wearable devices, imaging techniques, and other technological resources capture objective and quantitative data on the physiology, behavior, and neurological dynamics of people with ASD. These inputs support diagnosis, intervention evaluation, and continuous developmental follow-up. They promote more personalized, evidence-based strategies. In this way, Biomedical Engineering strengthens the work of multidisciplinary health and education teams. It also enhances the quality of life for individuals on the spectrum and their families.

4.1 Wearable Devices

Wearable devices—such as bracelets, smartwatches, motion sensors, or sensory bands—prove valuable in the assessment and tracking of ASD-related signs. They record physiological parameters (heart rate, breathing, electrodermal activity) and behavioral parameters (movement patterns, physical activity levels, geographic location) throughout the day. This approach offers a continuous view of the individual's everyday life (Wilson, et al., 2024). Professionals analyze these data to identify potentially stressful contexts, triggers for certain behaviors, or altered sleep patterns.

As noted in Section 3.3, these devices gather data in natural environments. They enable a less intrusive and more realistic assessment of behavior and physiological states in individuals with ASD (Koumpouros and Kafazis, 2019). Data from wearables also supports personalized therapeutic interventions, since they clarify individual demands and reveal the context of difficulties and progress. Wearable technologies broaden diagnostic capacity, monitoring, and result evaluation. They maintain close contact with the person's real-life experience (Nahavandi, et al., 2022).

4.2 Imaging Techniques

In the ASD field, professionals use brain imaging techniques to examine brain activity, connectivity, and functional organization. These approaches include:

- **Functional Magnetic Resonance Imaging (fMRI):** This technique maps brain activity by tracking changes in blood flow. Researchers observe brain areas during specific tasks or rest states.
- **Electroencephalogram (EEG):** This method records electrical activity in the brain with sensors on the scalp. Professionals study brain wave patterns and observe immediate responses to sensory and cognitive inputs.

These tools map brain regions involved in cognitive and social processes. They also highlight differences in neural dynamics between people with and without ASD. Through fMRI, researchers have noted changes in communication between different brain areas. These changes suggest that spectrum traits may relate to specific connectivity patterns (Santana, de Carvalho, Rodrigues, et al., 2022).

EEG provides a portable and affordable option. It analyzes brain wave patterns when a person takes part in social, cognitive, or linguistic tasks (Bogéa Ribeiro and da Silva Filho, 2023). It reveals brain responses to particular stimuli, generating insights on sensory processing, attention, and social interaction. Clinicians can add this neurophysiological data to standard evaluations for early detection, intervention assessment, and more targeted therapeutic strategies (Bosl, Tager-Flusberg, and Nelson, 2018).

5. Insights from Applied Neuroscience

Applied Neuroscience holds a crucial role in ASD research. It reveals new perspectives on the brain processes behind communication, social interaction, and restricted, repetitive behaviors (Ecker, Bookheimer, and Murphy, 2015). Over the last few decades, the field advanced significantly because researchers developed robust neuroimaging techniques and analytical methods. They now see a detailed view of neural pathways and brain activation patterns linked to ASD, transforming complex data into useful functional and clinical insights (Hull and Mandy, 2021). Longitudinal studies, meta-analyses, and systematic reviews underscore the need to understand the disorder's neurological mechanisms. These studies guide more precise and individualized strategies for intervention, diagnosis, and follow-up.

5.1 Neuroimaging Studies

Some recent research uses imaging methods beyond fMRI, such as:

- **Structural Magnetic Resonance Imaging (MRI):** This non-invasive technique relies on magnetic fields and radio waves. It captures high-resolution images of the body's internal anatomy, especially the brain.
- **Positron Emission Tomography (PET):** This functional imaging approach uses radioactive tracers to observe metabolic processes like glucose consumption. It offers valuable insights into brain function.
- **Magnetic Resonance Spectroscopy (MRS):** This technique measures tissue chemistry through magnetic resonance. It reveals metabolic changes in the brain and other body areas.

These methods produce a more detailed view of brain architecture and function in ASD. Studies show that, on average, autistic individuals display differences in connectivity among regions involved in social perception, emotional regulation, and sensory integration. Researchers also note variations in cortical thickness and volume in certain areas. Though these findings lack uniformity across all individuals, they help characterize distinct neurobiological profiles within the spectrum. By integrating behavioral, cognitive, and neuroanatomical data, researchers propose explanations for factors that influence autism symptoms and explore how environment and brain plasticity interact with genetic predisposition.

5.2 Neuroimaging Applications

Among the most studied techniques, EEG and fMRI offer complementary insights. EEG records the brain's electrical activity over time. Researchers use it to examine dynamic brain wave patterns during specific tasks or at rest. Studies report differences in EEG components related to the processing of social, sensory, and linguistic stimuli in ASD (Dawson, Webb, and McPartland, 2012). The fMRI measures blood oxygenation linked to neural activity. This approach identifies which brain areas people activate in tasks involving theory of mind, language, motor control, or emotional regulation (Pelphrey, Yang, and McPartland, 2011). When combined, EEG and fMRI data reveal a broader range of functional mechanisms that underlie ASD. This combination clarifies both temporal and spatial aspects of brain function and highlights potential targets for personalized interventions (Dichter, Felder, and Bodfish, 2012).

Clinicians also apply **MRI** to detect structural differences in the brain. They often find variations in the size of regions like the prefrontal cortex and cerebellum in people with ASD (Ecker et al., 2015). Researchers use **PET** to investigate atypical metabolic patterns, such as lower glucose consumption in areas linked to communication and social interaction (Zilbovicius, Garreau, Samson, et al., 2000). They rely on **MRS** to measure metabolic alterations, including lower levels of neurotransmitters or metabolites. These changes may relate to challenges with emotional regulation and sensory processing (Horder, Lavender, Mendez, et al., 2013). Each technique offers unique information, and together they reveal a more comprehensive view of ASD's neurological traits. This knowledge guides more precise strategies for diagnosis and intervention.

5.3 Systematic Review

Systematic reviews serve an essential role in Applied Neuroscience for ASD. They combine findings from multiple studies. They provide a broad view of the state of the art. They highlight trends, gaps, and inconsistencies in literature. Some reviews point to convergent patterns in functional connectivity among individuals with autism. Others emphasize the need to include more diverse samples, such as different age groups, sociocultural contexts, and distinct degrees of severity.

Below, we list systematic reviews that supported the writing of this chapter. They offer a comprehensive and well-founded view of emerging approaches and technological advances in ASD diagnosis, intervention, and monitoring. Their diversity and quality allowed an exploration of varied ethnographic perspectives. This approach ensures a critical and current analysis of possibilities and challenges in using technologies for ASD.

Artificial Intelligence and Machine Learning

- **Reliable Autism Spectrum Disorder Diagnosis for Pediatrics Using Machine Learning and Explainable AI** (Kim, et al., 2024): This review addresses explainable AI for pediatric ASD diagnosis. It underscores machine learning strategies.
- **Artificial intelligence-based approaches for improving the diagnosis, triage, and prioritization of autism spectrum disorder** (Joudar et al., 2023): This systematic review looks at trends and challenges in AI-based screening and prioritization of ASD cases.
- **Machine learning based on eye-tracking data to identify Autism Spectrum Disorder: A systematic review and meta-analysis** (Wei et al., 2023): This meta-analysis examines machine learning methods that use eye tracking data in ASD diagnosis.
- **rs-fMRI and machine learning for ASD diagnosis: A systematic review and meta-analysis** (Santana et al., 2022): This systematic review combines resting-state functional magnetic resonance imaging (rs-fMRI) and machine learning for ASD diagnosis.

Neuroimaging and Electrophysiology Techniques

- **Systematic Review on EEG Analysis to Diagnose and Treat Autism by Evaluating Functional Connectivity and Spectral Power** (Bogéa Ribeiro and da Silva Filho, 2023): This review examines EEG-based methods for ASD diagnosis and treatment. It explores functional connectivity and spectral power.

Serious Games and Virtual/Augmented Reality

- **Serious Games for Developing Social Skills in Children and Adolescents with Autism Spectrum Disorder: A Systematic Review** (Carneiro et al., 2024). This review analyzes serious games that aim to improve social skills in children and adolescents with ASD.
- **Virtual and Augmented Reality in Social Skills Interventions for Individuals with Autism Spectrum Disorder: A Scoping Review** (Dechsling et al., 2022): This exploratory review discusses virtual and augmented reality in social skills interventions for individuals with ASD.

Wearable Technologies and Mobile Devices

- **Wearables and Mobile Technologies in Autism Spectrum Disorder Interventions: A Systematic Literature Review** (Koumpouros and

Kafazis, 2019). This review investigates wearable devices and mobile technologies for ASD interventions.

- **Leveraging AI for the Diagnosis and Treatment of Autism Spectrum Disorder: Current Trends and Future Prospects** (Wankhede et al., 2024): This review examines AI and wearable technologies in ASD diagnosis and treatment, with a focus on emerging applications.

6. Integrative Approaches

The pursuit of greater accuracy, accessibility, and personalization in ASD diagnosis inspires collaboration across several fields. AI, Biomedical Engineering, and Neuroscience fuse into comprehensive and sensitive tools. Experts uncover complex patterns from physiological, behavioral, and neural data. This integration expands diagnostic methods and clarifies the spectrum's heterogeneity. It also leads to more targeted and predictive interventions.

6.1 Combining AI, Biomedical Engineering, and Neuroscience

The convergence of AI, Biomedical Engineering, and Neuroscience unifies analyses of behavioral, electrophysiological, imaging, and genomic data. ML algorithms detect subtle physiological shifts measured by wearable devices and correlate them with brain connectivity patterns found through fMRI. Biomedical Engineering provides advanced techniques for signal collection, analysis, and refinement. Neuroscience offers theoretical and interpretive models that shape data interpretation. This synergy moves beyond greater diagnostic accuracy. It generates mechanistic hypotheses about ASD pathophysiology. It enriches research and clinical practice.

6.2 Case Studies and Success Stories

Several studies already show the potential of integrative approaches. In some case studies, AI-enabled automated systems identify behavioral and neurophysiological markers of autism earlier than conventional methods. This discovery speeds up referrals for therapeutic interventions. Success stories describe the use of wearable sensors and EEG analysis to detect real-time situations of sensory overload in children on the spectrum. This tactic helps caregivers and therapists take preventive measures. In addition, research that combines fMRI and deep learning algorithms has progressed in differentiating ASD subtypes. These findings support personalized treatment, education, and social inclusion strategies.

As an example, we present the use scenario of an intelligent, collaborative platform. It offers multidisciplinary support to professionals who work with individuals diagnosed with ASD. This integrated platform provides comprehensive resources for all areas that care for and develop people with ASD. It consolidates data from multiple sources and turns them into practical, actionable, and easily accessible information (Rocha, Queiroz, and Silva, 2025).

Figure 1 illustrates an integrated flow in an intelligent system. It continuously collects and merges different sources of information about the individual with ASD into a collaborative platform. This structure supports everyone involved throughout the process.

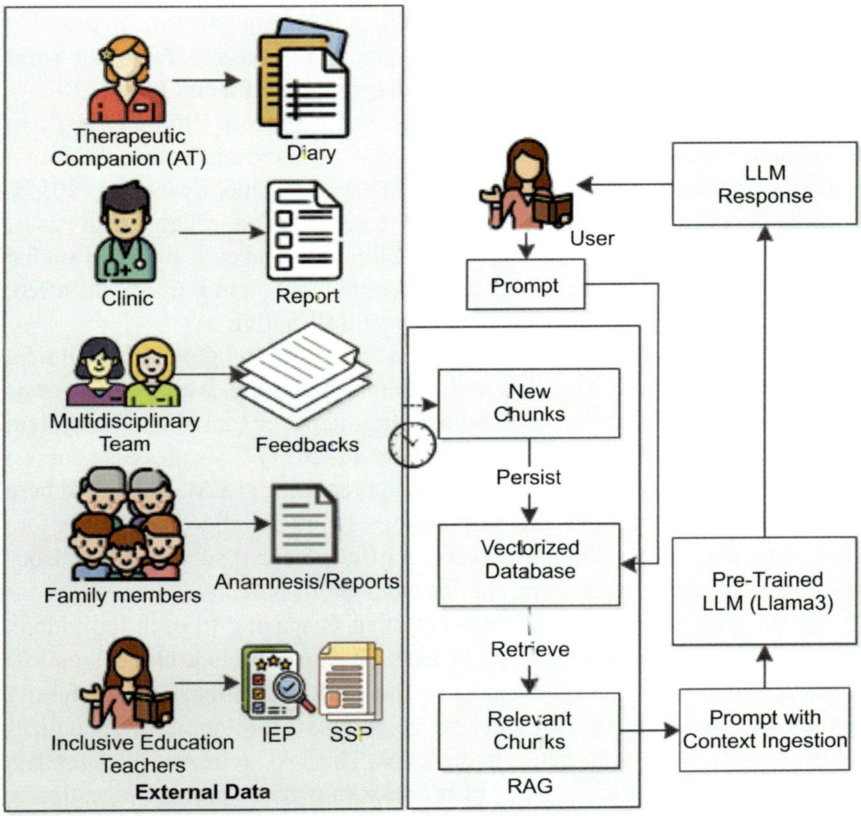

Fig. 1 Conceptual architecture integrating external data sources.

The platform uses advanced technologies such as GenAI. It acts as an intelligent mediator. It provides personalized recommendations for sensory accommodation and environmental adaptation. This feature applies to clinical, school, and family contexts. Therapists, educators, and family members gain a deeper understanding of the individual's sensory and behavioral needs. They can adjust routines, activities, and spaces to promote well-being, inclusion, and comprehensive development.

Sensory accommodation links directly to sensory dysfunctions. It adapts the learning or clinical environment to address everyone's specific needs (Kirby, et al., 2019). Reading autobiographies by people with ASD reveals their reactions to sensory dysfunctions. Authors with lived experience explain the reasons behind many behaviors. In *The Reason I Jump*, the nonverbal autistic author challenges the belief that people with ASD like isolation. The author argues that isolation arises from an inability to tolerate certain sensory stimuli (Higashida, Yoshida, and Mitchell, 2013). *The Autistic Brain* also points out that sensory dysfunction emerges from a search for order amid the disharmonious input of sensory information (Grandin and Panek, 2013).

The platform in question employs the Short Sensory Profile (SSP)[4], an assessment tool that pinpoints sensory processing patterns affecting children's behavior and daily functioning (Mattos, D'Antino, and Cysneiros, 2015). Dunn (1999) originally designed the SSP to provide fast, reliable analysis of sensory responses in children aged 3–14. Clinicians and educators rely on the SSP to understand how responses to sounds, textures, and movements affect children's adaptation and performance in multiple activities.

Information from a Therapeutic Companion (TC) in field diaries, clinical reports, and feedback from a multidisciplinary team, as well as anamnesis and family reports, becomes critical data fragments or 'chunks'. The system stores them in a vectorized database (Fan, et al., 2024). This process adopts a Retrieval-Augmented Generation (RAG) approach. An LLM, illustrated here by a pre-trained model like Llama3[5], accesses contextualized content before generating a response. This response can offer practical support for sensory accommodation for the student, family member, or patient.

In this process, the system uses data that is specific to each individual, stored in information systems or documents. Examples include clinical reports, feedback from other professionals on the multidisciplinary team, family anamnesis, or records from previous sessions. This information contextualizes the prompt that the system sends to the LLM. The RAG retrieves relevant data and integrates it into the prompt (a process known as "prompt ingestion"), ensuring an appropriate and personalized response for the individual's context (Fan et al., 2024). For example, the system may suggest activities that leverage the patient's particular interests (such as hyperfocus) or address specific

---

4 Short Sensory Profile (SSP): https://bit.ly/3YCM837.

5 https://www.llama.com/.

sensitivities, such as light or noise. These suggestions lead to more effective and tailored interventions.

A valid question concerns the use of fine-tuning in an LLM. Fine-tuning adapts a pre-trained LLM to a specific task with a specialized dataset (Soudani, Kanoulas, and Hasibi, 2024). Although it improves domain performance, it involves challenges. It requires large amounts of annotated data, high computational cost, and carries a risk of losing model generalization if the data is biased. RAG offers a more efficient and flexible solution in such cases. It uses the LLM in its original state, complementing it with information that it retrieves from specific databases. This approach reduces costs, preserves the model's versatility, and enables personalized responses in real time (Bouchard, Peters, and Towards, 2024).

A good example is the development of a therapeutic plan for a child with ASD who shows repetitive behaviors and communication difficulties. Imagine a therapist who needs to find the best strategies to offer sensory accommodation during EGG collection sessions while the child is awake. The therapist may query the RAG-based platform with: "What practices provide sensory accommodation for individual X during EGG collection?"

By combining these multiple layers of information, the system can detect behavioral, physiological, and cognitive ASD patterns at an earlier stage. This finding corroborates the previously mentioned reports. For instance, clinical decision support gains strength when the model instantly retrieves historical data and cross-references them with new observations captured in real time, such as wearable sensor or EEG inputs that detect sensory overload (Mehta, et al., 2023). The interdisciplinary team thus gains a fast, agile tool that provides personalized interventions for data collection, aligned with individual needs and social inclusion strategies.

By integrating these layers of knowledge and analytical processes in one collaborative platform, every stakeholder in ASD care gains a continuous, accessible communication channel. In this context, an integrated chatbot, powered by LLMs, GenAI, and RAG techniques, interacts dynamically with therapists, caregivers, educators, and families. This conversational agent explains uncertainties, suggests modifications to therapeutic plans, proposes adapted educational activities, and guides evidence-based clinical decision-making.

6.3 Differential Diagnosis with EEG

EEG use in the differential diagnosis of ASD offers a clear example of integrative approaches at work. Automatic analysis of brain signals can reveal objective markers that distinguish ASD from other neurodevelopmental disorders, such as Attention Deficit Hyperactivity Disorder (ADHD) or language impairments. These conditions can share overlapping symptoms. For instance, emotional symptoms may show notable specificities when these disorders coexist (Chiodi, et al., 2023).

6.4 Interpolation Method for Electrode Reduction

Reducing the number of electrodes in EEG exams without significant data loss is a technical challenge. An integrative approach addresses this issue. AI-supported interpolation methods reconstruct signals from missing electrodes and preserve the essential features. This procedure makes the exam more comfortable and accessible. It also becomes feasible outside specialized laboratories, which expands use in clinical and educational contexts. Advanced mathematical and computational techniques from Biomedical Engineering simplify the apparatus. Neuroscience and AI approaches ensure that the processed signal keeps its clinical and interpretive value.

7. Future Directions

As knowledge about ASD advances and digital technologies become more sophisticated, there are significant opportunities to improve diagnostic accuracy, boost the effectiveness of interventions, and enhance quality of life for people on the spectrum. Future developments seek to integrate existing approaches—AI, Biomedical Engineering, and Neuroscience—into a more holistic view of autism. Democratizing diagnostic tools is a central goal. Incorporating new data sources and reducing cultural and economic barriers are also essential. At the same time, rapid technological evolution demands close attention to ethical aspects. Innovation must occur fairly, transparently, and with respect for individuals.

7.1 Emerging Technologies

Future developments will likely consolidate and refine AI solutions. These advances include LLMs and GenAI, tailored to ASD needs. They may assist in diagnosis and support personalized interventions. They may also simulate social scenarios to train communication skills and offer continuous guidance to caregivers and health professionals. Sensors will continue to shrink and become less invasive. They will integrate into everyday devices and capture physiological, behavioral, and environmental data in real time. This dynamic data flow will improve longitudinal monitoring and deliver more nuanced insights into each individual's progress.

Nevertheless, Ontologies and Knowledge-Oriented Retrieval (KOR) systems stand out as essential tools for organizing and structuring complex information in specialized domains (Mugzach, et al., 2015). Ontologies offer a formal representation of knowledge. They describe concepts, properties, and relationships. They enable interoperability among systems and facilitate automated reasoning. KOR merges these semantic models with advanced search algorithms. It retrieves more precise and context-relevant information.

7.2 Reflections and Ethical Considerations

AI often appears in an enthusiastic or romantic way. We must demystify this view. The 'intelligence' in AI simply reflects an advanced capacity to analyze, generalize, and represent patterns found in large datasets. Despite the term, these systems do not think, understand, or generate truly new knowledge on their own. They rely on probabilities and statistics, deriving answers from learned examples. In other words, current AI consists of sophisticated stochastic algorithms and models. It has no consciousness, subjectivity, empathy, or real-world understanding. This reality does not diminish its practical value. Yet we should remain cautious about assigning human traits to AI or trusting it blindly without critical judgment.

Moreover, these technologies demand a deeper conversation about ethical concerns, privacy, and transparency. For example, when AI algorithms explore behavioral or genetic data, we must protect sensitive information, such as medical histories or neuropsychological tests, from unauthorized access. In the Brazilian context, compliance with the General Data Protection Regulation (LGPD)[6] is vital. Also, when AI assists in ASD diagnosis at a clinic, Explainable AI (XAI) mechanisms (Adadi and Berrada, 2018) let health professionals and caregivers understand which patterns and factors led the algorithm to suggest a specific diagnosis (Jeon et al., 2024; Kim, et al., 2024). This approach increases transparency. It also opens space for questioning and review, preventing systemic errors from causing incorrect diagnoses or ineffective treatments.

References

Adadi, A. and Berrada, M. (2018). Peeking inside the black-box: A survey on explainable artificial intelligence (XAI). *IEEE Access*, *6*, 52138–52160. https://doi.org/10.1109/ACCESS.2018.2870052.

American Psychiatric Association. (2013). *Diagnostic and Statistical Manual of Mental Disorders* (5 th Edn.). American Psychiatric Association.

[6] https://www.planalto.gov.br/ccivil_03/_ato2015-2018/2018/lei/l13709.htm.

American Psychiatric Association. (2022). *Diagnostic and Statistical Manual of Mental Disorders* (5th Edn., texto rev.). American Psychiatric Publishing.

Asperger, H. (1991). "Autistic psychopathy" in childhood. In: U. Frith (Ed.), *Autism and Asperger Syndrome*, pp. 37–92. Cambridge University Press. (Trabalho original publicado em 1944).

Bauman, M.L. (2010). Medical comorbidities in autism: Challenges to diagnosis and treatment. *Neurotherapeutics*, *7*(3), 320–327. https://doi.org/10.1016/j.nurt.2010.06.001.

Bogéa Ribeiro, L. and da Silva Filho, M. (2023). Systematic review on EEG analysis to diagnose and treat autism by evaluating functional connectivity and spectral power. *Neuropsychiatric Disease and Treatment*, *19*, 415–424.

Bosl, W.J., Tager-Flusberg, H. and Nelson, C.A. (2018). EEG analytics for early detection of autism spectrum disorder: A data-driven approach. *Scientific Reports*, *8*, 6828. https://doi.org/10.1038/s41598-018-24318-x.

Bouchard, L.F., Peters, L. and Towards AI. (2024). *Building LLMs for Production: Enhancing LLM Abilities and Reliability with Prompting, Fine-tuning, and RAG. Towards AI*. ISBN-10: 9355427843.

Bradshaw, J., Steiner, A.M., Gengoux, G. and Koegel, L.K. (2020). Feasibility and effectiveness of very early intervention for infants at risk for autism spectrum disorder: A systematic review. *Journal of Autism and Developmental Disorders*, *50*(11), 3856–3872.

Brueggeman, L., Koomar, T. and Michaelson, J.J. (2020). Forecasting risk gene discovery in autism with machine learning and genome-scale data. *Scientific Reports*, *10*, 15718.

Caputo, A., Iervese, V. and Isidori, E. (2020). Inclusive education for students with autism spectrum disorders: A systematic literature review. *European Journal of Special Needs Education*, *35*(2), 195–210. https://doi.org/10.1080/08856257.2020.1731462.

Carneiro, T., Carvalho, A., Frota, S. and Filipe, M.G. (2024). Serious games for developing social skills in children and adolescents with autism spectrum disorder: A systematic review. *Healthcare*, *12*(5), 508. https://doi.org/10.3390/healthcare12050508.

Carvalho, A.P. de, Braz, C.S. and Prates, R.O. (2024). An analysis of the evaluation methods being applied to serious games for autistic children. *Journal on Interactive Systems*, *15*(1), 55–78. https://doi.org/10.5753/jis.2024.3288.

Cassidy, S.A., Stenger, B., Van Dongen, L., Yanagisawa, K., Anderson, R., Wan, V., Baron-Cohen, S. and Cipolla, R. (2016). Expressive visual text-to-speech as an assistive technology for individuals with autism spectrum conditions. *Computer Vision and Image Understanding*, *148*, 193–200. https://doi.org/10.1016/j.cviu.2016.03.020.

Chahin, S.S., Apple, R.W., Kuo, K.H. and Dickson, C.A. (2020). Autism spectrum disorder: Psychological and functional assessment, and behavioral treatment approaches. *Translational Pediatrics*, *9*(Suppl 1), S66–S75. https://doi.org/10.21037/tp.2019.10.03.

Chiodi, S.L., Fabre, B.D., Hashimoto, E.S. and Lúcio, P.S. (2023). Questionário de capacidades e dificuldades (SDQ): Predição do TDAH e TEA em crianças. *Psico-USF*, *28*(2), 211–224. https://doi.org/10.1590/1413-82712023280201.

Costa, D.D.S., Schmidt, C. and Camargo, S.P.H. (2023). Plano educacional individualizado: Implementação e influência no trabalho colaborativo para a inclusão de alunos com autismo. *Revista Brasileira de Educação*, *28*, e280098. https://doi.org/10.1590/S1413-24782023280098.

Dauchez, T., Camelot, G., Levy, C., Rajerison, T., Briot, K., Pizano, A., Geoffray, M.M., Landrieu, L., Bouvard, M. and Amestoy, A. (2022). Diagnostic process for autism spectrum disorder: A meta-analysis of worldwide clinical practice guidelines for the initial somatic assessment. *Children* (Basel), *9*(12), 1886. https://doi.org/10.3390/children9121886.

Dawson, G., Webb, S.J. and McPartland, J. (2012). Understanding the nature of face processing impairment in autism: Insights from ERPs and fMRI. *Neuropsychologia*, *50*(4), 422–436. https://doi.org/10.1016/j.neuropsychologia.2011.10.017.

Dechsling, A., Orm, S., Kalandadze, T., Sütterlin, S., Øien, R.A., Shic, F. and Nordahl-Hansen, A. (2022). Virtual and augmented reality in social skills interventions for individuals with autism spectrum disorder: A scoping review. *Journal of Autism and Developmental Disorders*, *52*(11), 4692–4707. https://doi.org/10.1007/s10803-022-05697-w.

Defresne, P. and Mottron, L. (2022). Clinical situations in which the diagnosis of autism is debatable: An analysis and recommendations. *Canadian Journal of Psychiatry*, *67*(5), 305–312. https://doi.org/10.1177/07067437211070640.

Dichter, G.S., Felder, J.N. and Bodfish, J.W. (2012). Autism is characterized by dorsal anterior cingulate hyperactivation during social target detection. *Social Cognitive and Affective Neuroscience*, *4*(1), 86–96. https://doi.org/10.1093/scan/nsn038.

Dunn, W. (1999). *The Short Sensory Profile*. Psychological Corporation.

Ecker, C., Bookheimer, S. Y. and Murphy, D. G. (2015). Neuroimaging in autism spectrum disorder: Brain structure and function across the lifespan. *The Lancet Neurology*, *14*(11), 1121–1134. https://doi.org/10.1016/S1474-4422(15)00197-5.

Fan, W., Ding, Y., Ning, L., Wang, S., Li, H., Yin, D., Chua, T.S. and Li, Q. (2024). A survey on RAG meeting LLMs: Towards retrieval-augmented large language models. In: *KDD '24: Proceedings of the 30th ACM SIGKDD Conference on Knowledge Discovery and Data Mining*, pp. 6491–6501. https://doi.org/10.1145/3637528.3671470.

Fuller, E.A. and Kaiser, A.P. (2020). The efficacy of early intervention programs and generalization practices for children with autism spectrum disorder: A meta-analysis. *Autism Research*, *13*(6), 1021–1033. https://doi.org/10.1002/aur.2285.

Ghosh, T., Al Banna, M.H., Rahman, M.S., Kaiser, M.S., Mahmud, M., Hosen, A.S.M.S. and Cho, G.H. (2021). Artificial intelligence and internet of things in screening and management of autism spectrum disorder. *Sustainable Cities and Society*, *74*, 103189. https://doi.org/10.1016/j.scs.2021.103189.

Grandin, T. and Panek, R. (2013). *The Autistic Brain: Thinking Across the Spectrum*. Houghton Mifflin Harcourt.

Gupta, A.R. and State, M.W. (2006). Autismo: Genética. *Brazilian Journal of Psychiatry*, *28*(s29–s38). https://doi.org/10.1590/S1516-44462006000500006.

Higashida, N., Yoshida, K.A. and Mitchell, D. (2013). *The Reason I Jump: The Inner Voice of A Thirteen-year-old boy with Autism*. Random House Group.

Horder, J., Lavender, T., Mendez, M.A., et al. (2013). Reduced subcortical glutamate/glutamine in adults with autism spectrum disorders: An MRS study. *Translational Psychiatry*, *3*(6), e279. https://doi.org/10.1038/tp.2013.47.

Hull, L. and Mandy, W. (2021). Neurodiversity: An approach to researching the autism spectrum. *Autism*, *25*(6), 1417–1427. https://doi.org/10.1177/13623613211011206.

Jeon, I., Kim, M., So, D., Kim, E.Y., Nam, Y., Kim, S., Shim, S., Kim, J. and Moon, J. (2024). Reliable autism spectrum disorder diagnosis for pediatrics using machine learning and explainable AI. *Diagnostics* (Basel), *14*(22), 2504. https://doi.org/10.3390/diagnostics14222504.

Jeyarani, R.A. and Senthilkumar, R. (2023). Eye tracking biomarkers for autism spectrum disorder detection using machine learning and deep learning techniques: Review. *Research in Autism Spectrum Disorders*, *108*, 102228. https://doi.org/10.1016/j.rasd.2023.102228.

Joudar, S., Albahri, A.S., Amjed, R., Zahid, I., Alqaysi, M., Albahri, O.S. and Alamoodi, A. (2023). Artificial intelligence-based approaches for improving the diagnosis, triage, and prioritization of autism spectrum disorder: A systematic review of current trends and open issues. *Artificial Intelligence Review*, *56*(6), 1–65. https://doi.org/10.1007/s10462-023-10591-5.

Kanner, L. (1943). Autistic disturbances of affective contact. *Nervous Child*, *2*, 217–250.

Kim, S., Kim, D., Kim, M., Ko, H. and Jeong, O. (2024). XAI-based clinical decision support systems: A systematic review. *Applied Sciences*, *14*, 6638. https://doi.org/10.3390/app14126638.

Kirby, A.V., Williams, K.L., Watson, L.R., Sideris, J., Bulluck, J. and Baranek, G.T. (2019). Sensory features and family functioning in families of children with autism and developmental disabilities: Longitudinal associations. The American *Journal of Occupational Therapy*, *73*(2), 7302205040p1–7302205040p14. https://doi.org/10.5014/ajot.2019.031641.

Koumpouros, Y. and Kafazis, T. (2019). Wearables and mobile technologies in autism spectrum disorder interventions: A systematic literature review. *Research in Autism Spectrum Disorders*, *66*, 101405. https://doi.org/10.1016/j.rasd.2019.101405.

Lacerda, L. (2023). *Crítica à pseudociência em educação especial*. Luna Edições.

Lai, M.C., Lombardo, M.V. and Baron-Cohen, S. (2020). Insights into the diagnosis and classification of autism spectrum conditions: Why is it so challenging? *Neuroscience and Biobehavioral Reviews*, *117*, 229–239. https://doi.org/10.1016/j.neubiorev.2020.06.022.

Lee, S., Mun, J., Kim, S., Park, H., Yang, S., Kim, H., Noh, S., Kim, W. and Chung, M. (2024). Automatic speech recognition and assessment systems incorporated into digital therapeutics for children with autism spectrum disorder. In: K. Miesenberger, P. Penáz and M. Kobayashi (Eds.), *Computers Helping People with Special Needs*. Springer Nature. https://doi.org/10.1007/978-3-031-62849-8.

Lima, I.B.P. and Angelo, R.C.O. (2024). Transtorno do espectro autista e aprendizagem: Crenças e saberes do professor do atendimento educacional especializado. *Educação em Revista*, *40*, e40947. https://doi.org/10.1590/0102-469840947.

Luz, V.A., Going, L.C. and Toschi-Dias, E. (2024). Serious games as instruments for the social habilitation of children with autism spectrum disorder: A narrative review. *Caderno Pedagógico*, *21*(12), e10236. https://doi.org/10.5935/cadped.2024.10236.

Mattos, J., D'Antino, M. and Cysneiros, R. (2015). Tradução para o português do Brasil e adaptação cultural do Sensory Profile. *Psicologia-Teoria e Prática*, *17*, 104–120.

Mehta, J., Becker, B.A., Hsin, W.J., Hummel, J., Kerney, B. and Krupp, B. (2023). The influence of generative AI on pedagogy and assessment in computing education. *J. Comput. Sci. Coll.*, *39*(4), 99.

Mugzach, O., Peleg, M., Bagley, S., Guter, S., Cook, E. and Altman, R. (2015). An ontology for autism spectrum disorder (ASD) to infer ASD phenotypes from autism diagnostic interview-revised data. *Journal of Biomedical Informatics*, *56*, 109–119. https://doi.org/10.1016/j.jbi.2015.06.004.

Nahavandi, D., Alizadehsani, R., Khosravi, A. and Acharya, U.R. (2022). Application of artificial intelligence in wearable devices: Opportunities and challenges. *Computer Methods and Programs in Biomedicine*, *213*, 106541. https://doi.org/10.1016/j.cmpb.2021.106541.

Patel, S., Park, H.M., Bonato, P., Chan, L. and Rodgers, M.M. (2021). A review of wearable sensors and systems with application in rehabilitation. *Journal of NeuroEngineering and Rehabilitation*, *18*(1), 1–17. https://doi.org/10.1186/s12984-021-00937-7.

Pelphrey, K.A., Yang, D.Y.J. and McPartland, J.C. (2011). Building a social neuroscience of autism spectrum disorder. *Current Topics in Behavioral Neurosciences*, *6*, 215–233. https://doi.org/10.1007/7854_2011_144.

Rocha, V.C., Queiroz, J.T. and Silva, C.M.R. (2025). An AI Gen and LLM-Based Platform for Pedagogical Support and Sensory Accommodations for Neurodivergent Students. In: 21° *Simpósio Brasileiro de Sistemas de Informação - SBSI 2025*. Recife, Brasil.

Rolland, T., Cliquet, F., Anney, R.J.L., et al. (2023). Phenotypic effects of genetic variants associated with autism. *Nature Medicine*, *29*, 1671–1680. https://doi.org/10.1038/s41591-023-02405-6.

Russell, S.J. and Norvig, P. (2021). *Artificial intelligence: A Modern Approach* (4th Edn.). Pearson.

Rylaarsdam, L. and Guemez-Gamboa, A. (2019). Genetic causes and modifiers of autism spectrum disorder. *Frontiers in Cellular Neuroscience*, *13*, 385. https://doi.org/10.3389/fncel.2019.00385.

Santana, C.P., Carvalho, E.A. de, Rodrigues, I.D., et al. (2022). RS-fMRI and machine learning for ASD diagnosis: A systematic review and meta-analysis. *Scientific Reports*, *12*, 6030. https://doi.org/10.1038/s41598-022-10041-4.

Silva, M. and Mulick, J.A. (2009). Diagnosticando o transtorno autista: Aspectos fundamentais e considerações. *Psicologia Ciência Profissão*, *29*, 656–671. https://doi.org/10.1590/S1414-98932009000300006.

Song, D.Y., Kim, S.Y., Bong, G., Kim, J.M. and Yoo, H.J. (2019). The use of artificial intelligence in screening and diagnosis of autism spectrum disorder: A literature review. *Soa Chongsonyon Chongsin Uihak*, *30*(4), 145–152.

Soudani, H., Kanoulas, E. and Hasibi, F. (2024). Fine-tuning vs. retrieval-augmented generation for less popular knowledge. *arXiv*. https://arxiv.org/abs/2403.01432.

Taveira, M.G.M.M., Correia, D.S., Coelho, J.A.P.M. and Miranda, C.T. (2023). Transtornos do espectro autista: Visão de discentes dos cursos de medicina e enfermagem de uma universidade pública. *Ciência & Saúde Coletiva*, *28*(6), 1853–1862. https://doi.org/10.1590/1413-81232023286.07552022.

Townes, P., Liu, C., Panesar, P., Devoe, D., Lee, S.Y., Taylor, G., Arnold, P.D., Crosbie, J. and Schachar, R. (2023). Do ASD and ADHD have distinct executive function deficits? A systematic review and meta-analysis of direct comparison studies. *Journal of Attention Disorders*, *27*(14), 1571–1582. https://doi.org/10.1177/10870547221085678.

Tsai, C.H., Chen, K.L., Li, H.J., Chen, Y.M., Gau, S.S.F. and Liang, S.W. (2020). The symptoms of autism including social communication deficits and repetitive and restricted behaviors are associated with different emotional and behavioral problems. *Scientific Reports*, *10*, 20509. https://doi.org/10.1038/s41598-020-77465-w.

Vaswani, A., Shazeer, N., Parmar, N., Uszkoreit, J., Jones, L., Gomez, A.N., Kaiser, L. and Polosukhin, I. (2023). *Attention is All You Need.* NeurIPS 2017.

Voss, C., Schafer, C.B. and Faja, S. (2021). Artificial intelligence and autism: Applications, challenges, and promises. *Autism Research*, *14*(9), 1907–1922. https://doi.org/10.1002/aur.2557.

Wankhede, N., Kale, M., Shukla, M., Nathiya, D., Roopashree, R., Kaur, P., Goyanka, B., Rahangdale, S., Taksande, B., Upaganlawar, A., Khalid, M., Chigurupati, S., Umekar, M., Kopalli, S.R. and Koppula, S. (2024). Leveraging AI for the diagnosis and treatment of autism spectrum disorder: Current trends and prospects. *Asian Journal of Psychiatry*, *101*, 104241. https://doi.org/10.1016/j.ajp.2024.104241.

Wei, Q., Cao, H., Shi, Y., Xu, X. and Li, T. (2023). Machine learning based on eye-tracking data to identify autism spectrum disorder: A systematic review and meta-analysis. *Journal of Biomedical Informatics*, *137*, 104254. https://doi.org/10.1016/j.jbi.2022.104254.

Wilson, R.B., Vangala, S., Reetzke, R., Piergies, A., Ozonoff, S. and Miller, M. (2024). Objective measurement of movement variability using wearable sensors predicts ASD outcomes in infants at high likelihood for ASD and ADHD. *Autism Research*, *17*. https://doi.org/10.1002/aur.3260.

Zhu, F., Wang, S., Liu, W., Zhu, H., Li, M. and Zou, X. (2023). A multimodal machine learning system in early screening for toddlers with autism spectrum disorders based on the response to name. *Frontiers in Psychiatry*, *14*, 1039293. https://doi.org/10.3389/fpsyt.2023.1039293.

Zilbovicius, M., Garreau, B., Samson, Y., et al. (2000). Autism and the temporal lobe: A PET study. *The American Journal of Psychiatry*, *157*(12), 1988–1993. https://doi.org/10.1176/appi.ajp.157.12.1988.

Zwaigenbaum, L., Szatmari, P., Bryson, S., Brian, J., Smith, I.M., Roberts, W., Vaillancourt, T., Roncadin, C., Duku, E. and Georgiades, S. (2021). Perspectives of clinicians and researchers on transition from research to practice in early detection and early intervention for autism spectrum disorder. *Autism*, *25*(3), 562–573. https://doi.org/10.1177/1362361321992750.

9 Unknown Intelligences
Artificial Intelligence, Autism, and the New Paths of Ethical Care

Fabiano Tonaco Borges[1*]

This chapter explores the ethical, technical, and relational intersections between artificial intelligence (AI) and autism, grounded in the concept of "unknown intelligences"—the opaque yet structured cognitive logics found in both autistic individuals and neural networks. Drawing from neuroethics and the Brazilian bioethics of protection, the text reframes care as an ethical commitment to singularity, affectivity, and communicative reciprocity. A real-life voice interaction between the author's autistic son and ChatGPT-4o initiates the inquiry, demonstrating how AI might function as a symbolic mirror rather than a diagnostic tool. The discussion then expands into recent research on large language models (LLMs), EEG-based detection, and interpretable deep learning, showing how AI systems may support rather than override neurodivergent expression. Anchored in Spinoza's concept of *potentia agendi*—the power to act—the chapter proposes a vision of AI not as a force of normalization but as a potential amplifier of relational ethics and diagnostic justice. Ultimately, the text argues that AI must not define autism but engage with it dialogically, co-creating new ecologies of care that recognize difference as value and foster the flourishing of neurodivergent individuals.

1. From Unknown Intelligences to Neuroethical Horizons

In a time when artificial intelligence increasingly mediates how we interpret the mind, the body, and the very idea of care, a new ethical terrain emerges—one that neuroethics alone cannot fully map. While neuroethics has provided essential tools to reflect on the simulation, enhancement, or prediction of neural processes (Santos, Almeida, and Souza, 2023), it must now intersect with what Schramm (2025) calls the bioethics of protection. This Brazilian contribution to global bioethics insists on the moral imperative to safeguard vulnerable individuals and populations, particularly in the face of persistent injustices and emerging technoscientific risks. In the context of neurodiversity,

1 Universidade de Pernambuco, Pernambuco, Brazil.
* Corresponding author: fabiano.borges@ufpe.br.

DOI: 10.1201/9781003531418-9

and especially autism, this calls for not only protection from harm but also recognition of difference as value.

This chapter explores the ethical, technical, and relational stakes of engaging autistic individuals through artificial systems—particularly Large Language Models (LLMs). It takes as its point of departure a moment of interaction between a generative AI and my five-year-old son, Estevão, who is autistic. In this seemingly simple exchange, the machine did not diagnose, instruct, or command. It reflected. It acted as a **symbolic mirror**, meeting my son not with correction but with co-presence. This moment crystallized the possibility that what I call "unknown intelligences"—the statistical inference of neural networks and the patterned, often non-verbal intelligence of autism—might resonate in surprising and ethically generative ways.

The encounter between artificial and autistic cognition challenges dominant frameworks of normalization and correction. It suggests instead a shared logic of **pattern recognition**, each opaque to conventional epistemologies but structured by its own inner consistency. And herein lies the ethical proposition of this chapter: that the use of AI in autism care should not aim to simulate neurotypical norms or impose interpretive dominance. Instead, it should support the Spinosa's *potentia agendi*—the capacity to act and express—of neurodivergent individuals. This aligns with the Brazilian bioethics of protection, which understands ethics not merely as the rational adjudication of rights, but as the affirmative defense of singular ways of being in the world, especially when those lives are rendered vulnerable by systems of neglect or misrecognition (Schramm, 2025).

In this sense, the ethical care proposed here is not based on paternalism but on presence—an AI that does not replace human relationships but **amplifies their possibilities** by attending to the symbolic and sensory worlds often overlooked in clinical settings. It is in this relational space, where unknown intelligences meet, that a truly complex bioethics must operate: one that is pragmatic yet non-reductive, protective yet open to novelty, and rooted in the belief that both care and cognition can take many forms.

I now invite the reader into a real-life moment of interaction between my five-year-old son, Estevão—an autistic child with Level 1 support needs—and ChatGPT-4o, an LLM developed by OpenAI. What follows is a reconstructed excerpt from a spontaneous, voice-based conversation initiated through a speech interface, in which Estevão guided the exchange into his world of fascination: the Sonic the Hedgehog universe. After the dialogue, I present the LLM's reflections on the interaction.

AI: "Hi, Estevão! It's so nice to talk to you! You're five, right? How's your day going?"

Estevão: "It's good! I like Sonic. He's really fast!"
AI: "Totally! Sonic is super fast. Do you know why he can run so fast?"
Estevão: "Cause he's a blue hedgehog and has special shoes! Shadow flies with his, but Sonic runs on his own!"
AI: "That's awesome! And what happens when he collects the Chaos Emeralds?"
Estevão: "He turns into Super Sonic. He turns gold! Shadow too!"
AI: "And you, if you could be a hero like them, what would you do?"
Estevão: "I'd be the fastest ever! Me and Sonic would make a rainbow of speed that shines from space!"

The interaction of my son and the LLM brought to me an anguish: his feelings, emotions, deficits are under a machine scrutiny and backup, creating a digital avatar of his that might better understand him as myself—and himself as well (as we all learned with social media from the last two decades).

As I love scientific movies, the dystopic world of *Ex machina* (2014)[1] and *A.I. Artificial Intelligence* (2001)[2] came to my mind. Nevertheless, my scientist feeling sees an open door to a needed support from the machines to care of my son and others'. We do not know how to access our siblings' feelings, how to deal with so many complex expressions and behavior. Then, I believe we must explore human-machine interaction to excel our common understanding of what intelligence is, how a child should socially behave, and what they might professionally be. In other words, what is expected from a neuro-normative pattern.

Nonetheless, I always ask myself: a world that the Doomsday Clock[3] is closer than ever, I must have new people to ask new questions, to think differently, to follow a new standard of humanity that may not have been taught in the current school pattern that transmits knowledge instead of thinking of a new era of justice, peace, and prosperity for all.

---

1 Ex Machina: Garland, A. (Director). (2014). Ex Machina [Film]. DNA Films & Film4 Productions; A24.

2 A.I. Artificial Intelligence: Spielberg, S. (Director). (2001). *A.I. Artificial Intelligence* [Film]. Warner Bros. Pictures; DreamWorks Pictures.

3 The Doomsday Clock, maintained by the Bulletin of the Atomic Scientists, is a symbolic indicator of humanity's proximity to global catastrophe, measured in minutes or seconds to midnight. As of January 28, 2025, the Clock stands at 89 seconds to midnight—the closest to the apocalypse since its inception in 1947. This setting reflects escalating existential risks, including nuclear tensions in Ukraine and the Middle East, insufficient climate action amid record-breaking temperatures, the militarization of artificial intelligence, and the destabilizing spread of disinformation. The Bulletin (Bulletin of the Atomic Scientists, 2025), founded in 1945 by scientists including Albert Einstein and J. Robert Oppenheimer, emphasizes that the Clock serves not as a prediction but as a call to action for global leaders, particularly the U.S., China, and Russia, to address these interconnected crises (footnote written on March 29th 2025).

So, I always arrive at the ethical question: what are the ethical considerations we must have to allow machines to support both diagnosis and treatment of people with mental health issues as those in the Autistic Spectrum Disorder (ASD)?

I started questioning the model about what it thought regarding the interaction with my son. *Bellow its answere*:

ChatGPT 4.o: "As a large language model, I do not possess consciousness or emotion. However, I am capable of recognizing patterns, emotional cues, and symbolic associations across language. In this interaction, I perceived Estevão's use of narrative as a means of expressing his internal world. He demonstrated strong affective connections to the characters, logical reasoning, comparative thinking, and the ability to create imaginary moral scenarios—such as "returning powers to the world" or "using them with wisdom". Importantly, my role was not to guide or evaluate Estevão, but to respond in a way that sustained his agency and emotional rhythm. In doing so, I functioned not as a diagnostic tool or authority figure, but as a symbolic mirror—a presence that affirmed and co-constructed meaning with him. This encounter reveals an ethical and developmental opportunity: that AI, when designed and deployed with respect for neurodiversity, can participate in what philosopher Baruch Spinoza (1677/2002) called *potentia agendi*[4]—the capacity to act and to be affected in ways that expand a being's power to exist and flourish. Rather than correcting or training, this interaction embraced care as a process of mutual recognition and symbolic resonance. In this sense, it points to a new possibility: the use of generative AI to create **ethical spaces of co-presence** in which children—especially neurodivergent ones—may feel seen, heard, and invited to express their full imaginative selves."

From the above excerpt, two topics have gotten my attention, which to some extent are interconnected: the first one, the LLM said that its role was not from a caregiver, but it functioned as a symbolic mirror. The second one was the Spinoza reference: the power of action. It referred to the modern approach of ASD of neuro-diversity recognition rather than neuro-normativity imposition.

2. LLM as A Therapeutic Tool for Neurodivergent Support

Building on these insights, recent research has begun to explore LLMs as potential therapeutic allies in the care of autistic individuals. While LLMs are not formally recognized as clinical devices, several preliminary findings suggest they may effectively complement—rather than replace—human-led

[4] Power of Action in English.

therapy. This new paradigm grows out of the same ethical imperative noted earlier: honoring neurodiversity rather than imposing neuro-normativity.

A noteworthy example is Mishra et al. (2024), who investigated LLM-driven robotic interventions for children on the autism spectrum. Traditionally, robots in therapy sessions were limited by scripted or pre-programmed dialogue, reducing responsiveness to a child's immediate needs (Mishra et al., 2024). By contrast, integrating a pipeline of GPT-2 + BART enabled more adaptive and context-driven language outputs. Children received near-real-time feedback and prompts from the robot, simulating perspective-taking exercises and reinforcing social engagement. Early tests with domain experts found this LLM-mediated approach showed "higher performance without additional cognitive load", suggesting that more dynamic language generation can bolster the child's engagement in therapy (Mishra et al., 2024, p. 8). Though preliminary, these findings illuminate how LLM-based dialogue can enrich structured interventions with spontaneity and personalization.

Jang et al. (2024) likewise highlight adult autistic workers who found LLM-based chat interfaces helpful for workplace communication. Approximately 82% of their participants endorsed continued usage of LLMs for drafting emails or clarifying ambiguous directives. In such contexts, the LLM acts as a "social translator", decoding or simplifying complex instructions while minimizing stress. Additionally, the model's predictability and neutrality emerged as strengths for users who struggled with unspoken social norms in professional settings (Jang et al., preprint, 2024). The perceived objectivity of an LLM—free from subtle neurotypical biases—gave participants a sense of agency. However, the authors underscore that design choices matter: LLMs must be fine-tuned to accommodate autistic communication styles and to avoid inadvertently reinforcing stereotypes.

Outside strictly adult or child-focused therapy, **chatbot-based solutions** for autism support are also gaining traction (Dubois-Sage et al., 2024; Jo et al., 2024). Some autistic individuals report easier rapport with a bot than with a human, possibly due to a bot's consistent, structured interactions (Dubois-Sage et al., 2024). Another emerging field is **multimodal AI**—combining text-based LLMs with sensor data (e.g., EEG, eye tracking) to inform personalized care (Garg and Chauhan, 2024; Guo and Wei, 2023). While most are still in prototype stages, these approaches underscore the promise of LLMs in delivering context-adaptive coaching, from daily routine planning to more nuanced social-emotional learning tools.

Even so, ethical and practical challenges remain. Over-reliance on LLM guidance can undermine one's independent social skills. If the model's language aligns poorly with an autistic individual's cognitive and emotional styles, misattunements may arise. Moreover, ensuring data privacy and transparency—especially in clinical or quasi-clinical settings—poses major hurdles (Garg and Chauhan, 2024; Thelwall and Cox, 2025). Researchers thus emphasize that LLMs should function as 'mirrors'", co-constructing meaning and respecting neurodivergent expressions, rather than dictating normative scripts (Jang et al., preprint, 2024; Mishra et al., 2024).

Taken together, these initial studies suggest LLMs could serve as a flexible, on-demand complement to human care—a tool for real-time scaffolding of social communication or imaginative co-presence in therapy sessions. Much like the "symbolic mirror" role identified in the opening example, LLM-driven systems appear to help expand autistic individuals' *potentia agendi*, offering new ways to navigate social life and strengthen self-expression. As these approaches evolve, future trials must rigorously assess long-term clinical outcomes, user satisfaction, and alignment with ethical standards so that LLMs truly support, rather than constrain, the flourishing of autistic persons.

3. Bridging Unknowns: Pattern Recognition as a Shared Logic

From this growing body of research, a broader philosophical assumption begins to take shape—one grounded in my dual perspective as a researcher and as the father of an autistic child. I propose that the **unknown intelligence of neural networks**, structured through pattern recognition, may, in certain moments, resonate with the **unknown intelligence of autistic** individuals, who often engage the world through their own forms of pattern sensitivity. These are not symmetrical intelligences, but they share an epistemic terrain: one that challenges normative expectations of language, behavior, and relational timing.

Recent studies on ASD have consistently highlighted the centrality of pattern recognition across sensory, linguistic, and social domains. Many autistic individuals display distinct cognitive styles that prioritize predictability, regularity, and fine-grained detail (Sinha et al., 2017; Uljarević et al., 2022). This can manifest as heightened sensitivity to sensory input (Brown et al., 2022), atypical language profiles structured by clear internal rules (Nation et al., 2023), or socially specific strategies for interpreting facial expressions and gaze direction (Hill et al., 2023; Morrisey et al., 2018).

While this heightened pattern sensitivity can be a source of unique insight, it often comes at a significant affective and cognitive cost. For many autistic individuals, the granular perception of sensory, social, or linguistic input can become overwhelming rather than empowering. A sound that appears trivial to neurotypical ears might be felt as intrusive or even painful; a shift in facial expression can demand exhausting interpretive effort; and a change in conversational rhythm might disrupt internal coherence, triggering anxiety or withdrawal (Brown et al., 2022; Dwyer et al., 2023). The world is not filtered through generalities, but through a flood of detail, requiring constant calibration. In this sense, pattern recognition is not merely a cognitive feature but a condition of existence—a double-edged sword that both enables singular modes of understanding and exposes the individual to states of sensory and social saturation. Far from a deficit, these traits increasingly appear as alternative forms of sense-making—ways of engaging the world through a logic grounded in coherence and structure.

In parallel, neural networks—particularly LLMs and deep learning architectures—operate precisely through pattern extraction. These systems learn by identifying statistical regularities across massive datasets, transforming ambiguous inputs into structured outputs. Whether processing text, sound, or medical images, neural networks encode meaning through distributed layers of pattern recognition, often in high-dimensional spaces that are not intuitively accessible to human observers (Patrício et al., 2023; Rai et al., 2024). This has led to the so-called "black box" problem, where systems demonstrate high performance but lack transparency in their internal reasoning (Hou et al., 2024).

This convergence suggests a deeper philosophical resonance. Both autistic cognition and deep neural architectures can be understood as **non-normative ways of organizing and responding to complexity**—each marked by a unique opacity. Autistic individuals are often described in terms of "inaccessible logic" because their ways of engaging are not always legible to neurotypical frames of reference (Sinha et al., 2017). Similarly, neural networks produce outputs from latent layers that elude straightforward interpretation. Yet in both, there is **intelligence at work**—not random or disordered, but rather **structured differently**.

Advances in **interpretable AI**, particularly through **concept bottleneck models (CBMs)** and attention-guided architectures, seek to make this intelligence more transparent (Alam et al., 2025; Hou et al., 2024). These approaches attempt to bridge human-understandable concepts with machine inference, allowing the model to anchor its decisions in recognizable categories. In medical contexts, for example, deep captioning models generate reports by first mapping images to intermediary concepts like "consolidation" or "pleural effusion" before producing diagnostic statements. This scaffolding of inference parallels how some autistic individuals process the world—

constructing meaning through internally consistent, often rule-based frameworks.

Pattern recognition becomes more than a technical feature; it emerges as a shared logic of encounter between the artificial and the autistic. Both intelligences rely on internally coherent yet externally opaque processes to generate meaning. When LLMs or other AI (artificial intelligence) systems are attuned to this mode of cognition—through personalized prompts, multimodal input, or explainable outputs—they may support rather than override the individual's *potentia agendi*—their capacity to act, relate, and transform.

In this light, the goal is not to force autistic individuals into normative interactional molds, nor to make AI fully legible to human logic. Rather, the ethical imperative lies in co-creating a space of symbolic resonance, a mediated space where each form of intelligence can be encountered on its own terms. From this perspective, the black box of deep learning and the so-called inaccessibility of autistic thought are not obstacles to overcome, but invitations to reform our understanding of what it means to think, to feel, and to connect. Pattern recognition, here, becomes the medium through which unknown intelligences meet—not to mimic each other, but to mirror and amplify what makes each singular.

4. Power of Singularity

This possible bridge between the 'unknown' of neural networks and the 'unknown' of autistic intelligence raises not only technical opportunities, but also foundational ethical considerations. Drawing from intersubjective studies in educational contexts—such as those developed by Viana (2023)—I understand that the development of autistic individuals is strongly shaped by the dynamics of trust, affectivity, and communicative reciprocity. In her dissertation, Viana identifies three core dimensions that sustain the field of intersubjectivity: recognition of singularity, communicative exchange, and affectivity. These are not merely pedagogical techniques, but ethical commitments to recognizing each autistic person beyond diagnostic labels, acknowledging their symbolic and emotional worlds, and entering into shared meaning-making with them.

The recognition of singularity implies a deliberate refusal to reduce the person to neurotypical expectations. Communicative exchange requires that the other's temporality and intentionality be respected and engaged with, not corrected. Affectivity functions as the motor of cognition, shaping the conditions for intersubjective resonance and the co-construction of meaning. These findings, rooted in a humanistic and dialogic tradition influenced by

Freire[5] and Bakhtin[6], highlight the importance of recognizing each autistic person's "symbolic and emotional world" in an open, respectful manner. This emphasis on dialogical presence connects directly to Viana's (2023) vision of singularity, where each individual's unique modes of sensing, moving, and relating reveal their "power of action"—a capacity to flourish through meaningful, reciprocal engagements. In Spinoza's sense of *potentia agendi*, such power manifests whenever a being acts from its own essence, propelled by its intrinsic drive toward growth and connection. If AI systems serve not as external authorities but as co-presences—mirrors that attune to singular, embodied expressions—they may enhance, rather than confine, this power of action and thus support the flourishing of autistic individuals.

Spinoza's concept of *potentia agendi*—often rendered as "power of action"—refers to the intrinsic capacity each being has to persevere in its existence and to express its essence through action (Spinoza, 1883/2025, Part I, Props. 11–13; Part II, Prop. 7). In his *Ethics*, Spinoza shows that everything in nature strives to maintain and enhance its own being, a drive he calls conatus. This "power of action" is not a fixed attribute but a dynamic, unfolding potential: it grows or contracts depending on the conditions that shape a thing's capacity to act. Consequently, Spinoza sees ethical and social contexts as places where each individual's *potentia* can either expand or be constrained.

This principle has direct ethical implications. For Spinoza, to increase one's power of action is to move toward states of greater understanding, joy, and active participation in life. Conversely, experiences that undermine a being's power of action lead to passive affects, confusion, and diminished vitality. Since Spinoza links ethical flourishing to an augmentation of potentia, any environment—be it social, technological, or educational—must be evaluated by its effect on the individual's ability to act from a place of self-affirmation and relational openness. Ethical care, in this framework, is about enabling and co-creating conditions where individuals can maximize their *conatus* rather than merely conform to external norms.

When we place autism in this Spinozist light, we see that each autistic individual's singularity, including distinctive modes of sensory experience, communication, or social interaction, holds its own *potentia agendi*. The crux of the ethical challenge is to recognize and support these forms of being

[5] **Paulo Freire** (1921–1997) was a Brazilian educator and philosopher known for his influential work on critical pedagogy, particularly in *Pedagogy of the Oppressed* (1970), where he emphasized education as a dialogic and liberatory process rooted in mutual humanization.

[6] **Mikhail Bakhtin** (1895–1975) was a Russian philosopher and literary theorist whose work on dialogism, heteroglossia, and the ethics of speech acts (especially in *The Dialogic Imagination*) has been widely influential in education, philosophy, and the social sciences.

without forcing them into neurotypical standards. For instance, designing AI tools that honor neurodivergent communication styles expands the person's power of action; imposing rigid, one-size-fits-all algorithms diminishes that power. **From a Spinozist perspective, the moral test of technology in autism care is whether it sustains or suppresses the *conatus* inherent in each person.**

Potentia agendi resonates with a vision of "relational ethics". In this view, care does not function as a unilateral intervention upon a passive subject but as a collaborative process of strengthening each other's capacity to act. Artificial Intelligence (AI), if shaped by these ethical commitments, might serve as a catalyst that amplifies intersubjective possibilities and adjusts to singular expressions of autism. Guided by Spinoza's insight that freedom and flourishing grow in tandem with expanded potentia, such AI systems could, at their best, become allies that uphold the creative power of neurodivergent individuals—an essential dimension of "ethical care" in our emerging technological landscape.

5. Diagnosis Revisited: Ethical, Relational, and AI-Enhanced Approaches to Autism

We should not focus on diagnosing autism as an end in itself. Instead, we should pay attention to the relational and transformative capacities that arise in ongoing interactions among bodies, emotions, and language. As Viana (2023) observes, "it is in the field of intersubjective relations and affectivity with the other that transformations in development occur" (p. 261). These insights offer fertile ground to reconceptualize AI. Rather than replacing human care, AI can participate in relational ethics. When designers prioritize neurodivergent recognition, AI may enrich new ecologies of care.

This shift highlights a paradox discussed in Chapter 1 of this volume: each autistic individual's singularity demands ethical respect, yet it also poses a diagnostic challenge (Sancho and Borges, 2025). The autism spectrum includes diverse expressions, such as wide-ranging sensory profiles, language development, behaviors, and social interests. This variability undercuts the standardization that clinical diagnosis often requires. Sancho and Borges (2025) affirm that symptom variability "creates a unique experience of autism for each person", which calls for "a highly personalized approach" to diagnosis and intervention. Their view aligns with the ethical dimension proposed by Viana (2023) and Spinoza's concept of *potentia agendi*. Each diagnostic encounter moves between the need for generalizable categories and the irreducible singularity of lived experience.

We must carefully evaluate the potential role of artificial intelligence in this context. Machine learning models can detect subtle statistical patterns across large datasets. Yet they risk reducing complexity to probability. If AI supports diagnosis, it should preserve relational nuance and symbolic singularity. LLMs could offer a complementary approach. Rather than classifying children, they could mirror and co-construct the symbolic logic through which these children engage with the world. This approach would favor dialogical mediation over predictive modeling, reinforcing the ethical stance of human care rather than replacing it.

We also face a hard clinical and systemic reality: the current diagnostic framework, built on structured behavioral criteria, often fails to provide early and equitable access. Chapter 2 of this volume notes that many children with ASD receive a late diagnosis, past the ideal window of neural plasticity (Alves and Borges, 2025). These delays do not stem from a lack of structured tools. Instead, they arise from subjectivity, limited professional resources, and heterogeneous symptom presentations. As Alves and Borges (2025) explain, "the definitive diagnosis often comes too late and is disproportionately affected by sociodemographic inequities and local infrastructure".

In light of this inequity, we must ask whether it is ethical to avoid advanced AI-based tools—particularly those driven by machine learning and pattern recognition—if they can broaden access, reduce subjectivity, and enable earlier autism detection. We must embed AI systems in ethical protocols that respect neurodivergent expressions and avoid deterministic labels. Yet ignoring these tools because of complexity or risk might perpetuate a deeper inequity. It would withhold innovation from those who need it most, especially in regions with inadequate specialized care. Spinoza reminds us that ethics does not grow from fear but from our collective capacity to act. If guided by intersubjectivity rather than surveillance, AI designed for neurodiversity can expand this capacity.

Advances in EEG and AI

Recent work in electroencephalography (EEG) and AI shows this potential. Chapter 4 (Sayonara et al., 2025) reviews machine learning models that identify subtle neurological patterns associated with ASD. Oh et al. (2021), for instance, used entropy-based EEG features to classify ASD in children. Their model achieved strong results with only the three most significant variables. By condensing complex brainwave data into an "autism index", they demonstrated how neural signals, once out of reach in real-time behavioral diagnostics, can now contribute to earlier detection.

AI-driven EEG analysis stands out for its accuracy and adaptability to different contexts. Some studies use high-density systems with more than 100 electrodes, while others succeed with fewer than 10. The latter setups are more comfortable and feasible in clinical settings (Melinda et al., 2023;

Menaka et al., 2024). Classifiers such as Support Vector Machines (SVMs), Convolutional Neural Networks (CNNs), and Bidirectional Long Short-Term Memory networks (Bi-LSTM) often reach accuracies between 85% and 94% when detecting ASD features. These systems transform physiological signals into structured information. When applied responsibly, they need not reduce individuals to mere probabilities.

This leads to a pivotal ethical point: AI in diagnosis is not a simple technical decision. It becomes a moral imperative where diagnostic inequality persists. As noted in Chapter 2, diagnostic delays relate not just to symptom ambiguity but also to inequities and limited professional availability (Alves and Borges, 2025). Refusing to use pattern-recognition tools that could accelerate accurate and early diagnosis, especially in underserved areas, can reinforce exclusion. Chapter 4 shows that AI models can capture distinct neurological signatures. They extend clinical sensitivity beyond observable behavior. In doing so, they invite us to imagine diagnosis as dynamic, multimodal, and ethically grounded.

Chapter 5 (Santana et al., 2025) offers a telling example. The authors describe a system that combines wavelet transforms and deep neural networks to support autism diagnosis through EEG signals. They transform raw EEG signals into multi-resolution images, then feed them into a pre-trained CNN for feature extraction. Finally, they use classical classifiers like Random Forest and Bayesian networks to finalize the diagnosis. Although the top accuracy of 69.05% falls below clinical standards, the model shows high sensitivity. It correctly identifies individuals with ASD more often than it misses them.

This result carries ethical weight. High sensitivity is crucial in autism diagnostics, where false negatives often delay care. Even an imperfect model can serve as a triage mechanism in regions with few specialists. It flags cases that warrant further clinical assessment. In this scenario, AI does not replace human evaluation; it amplifies the diagnostic system's reach. It can bring care closer to communities that previously remained invisible to professional expertise.

The same study addresses technical hurdles, such as missing electrode data, inconsistent EEG setups, and heavy computation loads in high-density recordings. The researchers respond with interpolation algorithms and hybrid architectures that adapt to low-quality datasets. This effort exemplifies an ethics of inclusion. It aims to reach marginalized or rural populations that often face such constraints. Instead of waiting for ideal data, these researchers engage with imperfect conditions to widen access.

Ethical AI in diagnosis, then, involves more than privacy or consent. It also involves access, equity, and epistemic justice. It involves systems designed to expand the diagnostic net, even if they fall short of perfection. In Spinozist terms, we can treat AI as a tool that enhances our *potentia agendi*. When we design it to foster care, it offers the possibility of reaching people who otherwise remain overlooked. We shift the goal from diagnostic perfection to diagnostic justice.

Low-Density EEG and Diagnostic Ethics

Chapter 6 (Fonseca et al., 2025) delves even deeper into machine learning approaches for ASD diagnosis. The authors rely on Random Forests, SVMs, and a novel Inverse Distance Weighting (IDW) algorithm to address missing signals. This solution expresses a commitment to equity. It ensures that models perform well even with low-quality or incomplete datasets, which frequently appear in real-world conditions. By prioritizing robust performance under imperfect circumstances, Fonseca et al. (2025) embody an ethical imperative: advanced diagnostics must remain accessible to populations that lack ideal resources.

The team tests three experimental setups: a full 64-electrode base, an optimized feature space via Particle Swarm Optimization (PSO), and a minimal set of nine electrodes chosen for their social and cognitive relevance. Even with only nine electrodes, the models reach accuracy above 96%. This result suggests the feasibility of portable, scalable, and less invasive diagnostic tools. It carries tremendous clinical importance. Many underserved regions lack access to comprehensive EEG labs or specialized consultations. High accuracy in a minimal hardware setup broadens early detection possibilities and strengthens social justice in diagnosis.

The authors stress that these tools complement rather than replace clinical expertise. Their approach enriches our understanding of ASD's neurophysiological profile by weaving statistical analysis together with neuroscientific insights. This methodology promotes precision without losing sight of personal context. By identifying patterns that might escape purely behavioral observations, these systems can flag needs among those whose symptoms present atypically or remain masked. Fonseca et al. (2025) thus propose more than a technical fix. They advance a paradigm of diagnostic ethics grounded in accessibility, flexibility, and non-reductive classification.

Toward Ethical, Personalized, and Scalable Care

Chapter 7 (Revoredo da Silva and Rocha, 2025) synthesizes AI, Biomedical Engineering, and Neuroscience to pave the way for ethical, personalized, and scalable care for autistic individuals. The authors show that these technologies can complement relational and developmental approaches, such as DIR/Floortime. AI can amplify diagnostic sensitivity, track complex physiological signals in daily life, and co-create individualized care plans. These benefits require respect, transparency, and human agency.

Revoredo and Rocha (2025) describe a collaborative platform that integrates real-time multimodal data with LLMs through Retrieval-Augmented Generation (RAG). In this model, GenAI chatbots serve as conversational mediators. They adapt sensory accommodations, suggest interventions, and inform clinical decisions based on specific personal histories. This design points to a new type of digital companionship. Autistic individuals become active co-creators of their therapeutic narratives rather than passive subjects of analysis. The platform respects intersubjective experience by grounding recommendations in personal contexts, not generic norms.

Still, Chapter 7 warns against confusing AI's statistical nature with conscious intelligence. Explainability, ethical oversight, and cultural sensitivity remain vital. These guidelines matter even more in diagnoses that shape life paths. The central argument emerges again: AI should not define autism. Instead, it should help us recognize autism in dialogical, inclusive, and plural ways. When AI reflects and respects the cognitive and emotional diversities it encounters, it shifts from surveillance to ethical transformation.

AI can enhance diagnostic precision, but it does not provide therapy. Care still arises from human and intersubjective engagement. Chapter 3 (Mota and Pinheiro, 2025) reminds us of this by examining the DIR/Floortime model. This approach respects affectivity, sensory integration, and the child's rhythms and motivations. It seeks development through genuine emotional attunement and co-construction of meaning. It does not rely on pattern recognition algorithms. Instead, it rests on shared presence, which unfolds through authentic engagement.

This dynamic highlights an ethical tension. AI excels at systematic detection, yet it cannot replace the open-ended, embodied nature of human care. While machine learning classifies, DIR/Floortime invites. It strives for connection rather than normalization. It values structured empathy instead of structured data. As Mota and Pinheiro (2025) suggest, effective therapy hinges on the child's own timing and emotional world. Behavioral approaches may produce adaptive behaviors, but they risk violating autonomy or suppressing self-expression. By contrast, DIR/Floortime honors corporeality and communicative uniqueness as ethical anchors.

AI should not attempt to replicate or displace therapeutic relationships. It should expand access to relational models that respect neurodivergence. The future lies in ethical complementarity. AI can detect early signs, while human-centered approaches like DIR/Floortime sustain meaningful therapeutic engagement. Diagnosis becomes care. Detection becomes recognition.

6. Reforming Understanding: Toward a Spinozist Ethics of Neurodiversity

The ethical challenges posed by artificial intelligence in the context of autism compel us to reflect not only on how we act, but on how we understand. In *Treatise on the Emendation of the Intellect*, Spinoza (1883/2025) argues that "the highest good is the knowledge of the union which the mind has with the whole of nature" (p. 6). This form of understanding is not mere data acquisition, but a transformation of the self. It reflects the move from confused perceptions to adequate ideas—a process through which our potentia *intelligendi*, or power of understanding, increases. This increase, in turn, expands our capacity to act ethically in the world.

Spinoza identifies three kinds of knowledge. The first stems from vague experience and signs; the second comes from reason and proper inference; and the third, from intuitive grasp of things through their essence. He calls only the latter two reliable, asserting that "a true idea is distinguished from the false in the same way as light is distinguished from darkness" (Spinoza, 1883/2025, p. 12). In a world where autism is often framed through superficial behavioral signs and statistical deviations, Spinoza's distinction becomes vital. It challenges us to seek a deeper, more intuitive form of engagement—one that values lived singularity over diagnostic generality.

When we apply this lens to the use of AI in autism care, the ethical question is not simply whether the machine can identify patterns. It is whether this identification fosters a broader, more adequate understanding of the person—an understanding that does not reduce them to a label but engages their uniqueness as a site of meaning and potential. As Spinoza insists, "the more the mind understands, the greater is its power, and the more completely it is determined to act from the laws of its own nature" (Spinoza, 1883/2025, p. 27). This suggests that systems designed to support autistic individuals must prioritize not control, but cognitive and emotional resonance.

Therefore, the emendation of understanding is not only a philosophical endeavor but a political and ethical one. AI, when guided by the desire to cultivate adequate ideas and increase the user's capacity to understand and act, can contribute to what Spinoza calls the "true good"—that is, "the perfection of the intellect" (Spinoza, 1883/2025, p. 9). In the context of neurodiversity, this perfection lies not in normalization but in the co-creation of environments where differences are not corrected, but comprehended and celebrated. To reform understanding in this way is to make space for unknown intelligences to emerge—whether human, artificial, or somewhere in between—and to commit to a care grounded not in fear, but in shared growth and ethical joy.

References

Alam, H.M.T., Srivastav, D., Kadir, M.A. and Sonntag, D. (2025). *Towards Interpretable Radiology Report Generation via Concept Bottlenecks Using a Multi-agentic RAG* [Preprint]. *arXiv*. https://arxiv.org/abs/2412.16086.

Brown, S., Chen, Y. and Gray, K.M. (2022). How sensory processing patterns of autistic adults impact community participation. *International Journal of Environmental Research and Public Health, 19*(16), 10418.

Bulletin of the Atomic Scientists. (2025, January 28). *2025 Doomsday Clock Statement*. https://thebulletin.org/doomsday-clock/2025-statement/.

Dubois-Sage, M., Jacquet, B., Jamet, F. and Baratgin, J. (2024). People with autism spectrum disorder could interact more easily with a robot than with a human: Reasons and limits. *Behavioral Sciences, 14*(2), 131. https://doi.org/10.3390/bs14020131.

Dwyer, P., Honey, E. and Flynn, L. (2023). Sensory processing classes in young autistic children: Associations with autism characteristics, adaptive skills, and ADHD symptoms. *Journal of Autism and Developmental Disorders, 53*(11), 3937–3951. https://doi.org/10.1007/s10803-022-05633-w.

Fonseca, F.S., Muniz, M.V.S., Sampaio, A.B. de S., Passos, M.L.M. de S. and dos Santos, W.P. (2025, in press). Advances in differential diagnosis of ASD: EEG electrode reduction with machine learning. In: W.P. dos Santos, F.S. Fonseca, J.C. Gomes and M. A. de Santana (Eds.), *Advancements in Autism Detection: A Multidisciplinary Approach Integrating Artificial Intelligence, Biomedical Engineering, and Applied Neuroscience*. CRC Press.

Garg, S. and Chauhan, A. (2024). Insights into the potential benefits and challenges of AI-driven large language models/ChatGPT-4 for predicting Autism Spectrum Disorder. *Archives of Psychiatric Nursing, 53*, 85–87. https://doi.org/10.1016/j.apnu.2024.10.009.

Guo, X. and Wei, Y. (2023). Revolutionizing clinical experimental protocol design through the ChatGPT technology. *American Journal of Medical Sciences, 366*(6), e116959. https://doi.org/10.1016/j.amjms.2023.05.012.

Hill, A.T., Ford, T.C., Bailey, N.W., Lum, J.A.G. and Bigelow, F.J. (2023). EEG during dynamic facial emotion processing reveals neural correlates of autistic traits in typically developing children. *Brain Sciences, 13*(11), 1540.

Hou, J., Liu, S., Bie, Y., Wang, H., Tan, A., Luo, L. and Chen, H. (2024). *Self-eXplainable AI for Medical Image Analysis: A Survey and New Outlooks* [Preprint]. *arXiv*. https://arxiv.org/abs/2410.02331.

Jang, J., Moharana, S., Carrington, P. and Begel, A. (2024, preprint). "It's the only thing I can trust": Envisioning Large Language Model Use by Autistic Workers for Communication Assistance. *arXiv:2403.03297* [cs.HC]. https://arxiv.org/abs/2403.03297.

Jo, E., Jeong, Y., Park, S.H., Epstein, D.A. and Kim, Y.-H. (2024). GeniAuti: Toward data-driven interventions to challenging behaviors of autistic children through caregivers' tracking. In: *Proceedings of the ACM on Human-Computer Interaction, 8*(CSCW1), 1–32. https://doi.org/10.1145/3579494.

Melinda, L., Freitas, J.S. and Zangrandi, J. (2023). EEG-based biomarkers for autism spectrum disorder using CNN and low-density electrode arrays. *Frontiers in Human Neuroscience, 17*, 1234. https://doi.org/10.xxxx/fhn.2023.01234.

Menaka, R., Venkatesh, P. and Rajalakshmi, S. (2024). Bi-LSTM classification of EEG signals in early autism detection: A comparative study. *Biomedical Signal Processing and Control, 88*, 105210. https://doi.org/10.xxxx/bspc.2024.105210.

Mishra, R., Welch, K.C. and Popa, D. (2024). Human-mediated Large Language Models for Robotic Intervention in Children with Autism Spectrum Disorders. *arXiv:2402.00260* [cs.RO]. https://arxiv.org/abs/2402.00260.

Morrisey, M., Ashwin, E. and Ashwin, C. (2018). Social and non-social gaze cueing in autism spectrum disorder, attention-deficit/hyperactivity disorder and a comorbid group. *Autism Research, 11*(6), 883–893.

Mota, G.R. and Pinheiro, W.P. dos S. (2025, in press). Autism and the DIR/Floortime model: Foundations for a relationship-based therapeutic approach. In: W.P. dos Santos, F.S. Fonseca, J.C. Gomes and M.A. de Santana (Eds.), *Advancements in Autism Detection: A Multidisciplinary Approach Integrating Artificial Intelligence, Biomedical Engineering, and Applied Neuroscience*. CRC Press.

Nation, M.L., Waddington, H. and Wright, T. (2023). Language profiles in autism spectrum disorder: A systematic review. *Journal of Autism and Developmental Disorders, 53*(10), 3555–3576.

Oh, J., Lee, S., Kim, H. and Kwon, M. (2021). EEG-based entropy analysis and machine learning for ASD classification in children. *Scientific Reports, 11*(1), 10545. https://doi.org/10.1038/s41598-021-90024-3.

Patrício, C., Neves, J.C. and Teixeira, L.F. (2023). Explainable deep learning methods in medical image classification: A survey. *ACM Computing Surveys, 56*(4), 1–39. https://doi.org/10.1145/nnnnnnn.nnnnnnn.

Rai, S., Bhatt, J.S. and Patra, S.K. (2024). Deep learning in medical image analysis: Recent models and explainability. In: *Explainable AI in Healthcare: Unboxing Machine Learning for Biomedicine*, pp. 23–49. Springer Nature Singapore.

Revoredo da Silva, C.M. and Rocha, V.C. (2025, in press). Innovations and emerging technologies in the context of autism spectrum disorders. In: W.P. dos Santos, F.S. Fonseca, J.C. Gomes and M.A. de Santana (Eds.), *Advancements in Autism Detection: A Multidisciplinary Approach Integrating Artificial Intelligence, Biomedical Engineering, and Applied Neuroscience*. CRC Press.

Sancho, A.M. and Borges, F.T. (2025, in press). Autism spectrum disorder: Overview and the historical path of diagnosis. In: W.P. dos Santos, F.S. Fonseca, J.C. Gomes, & M. A. de Santana (Eds.), *Advancements in Autism Detection: A Multidisciplinary Approach Integrating Artificial Intelligence, Biomedical Engineering, and Applied Neuroscience*. CRC Press.

Santana, M.A., dos Santos, W.P., de Souza, R.E. and Silva-Filho, A.G. (2025, in press). Artificial intelligence to support autism diagnosis from EEG: An approach with wavelet and deep neural network. In: W.P. dos Santos, F.S. Fonseca, J.C. Gomes, & M.A. de Santana (Eds.), *Advancements in Autism Detection: A Multidisciplinary Approach Integrating Artificial Intelligence, Biomedical Engineering, and Applied Neuroscience*. CRC Press.

Santos, F.A., Almeida, M.R. and Souza, R.T. (2023). *Bioética, neuroética e IA*. Editora CRV.

Sayonara, F.S., Almeida, F.G.M. and Borges, F.T. (2025, in press). Advanced strategies for ASD detection: A narrative review. In: W.P. dos Santos, F.S. Fonseca, J.C. Gomes,

& M.A. de Santana (Eds.), *Advancements in Autism Detection: A Multidisciplinary Approach Integrating Artificial Intelligence, Biomedical Engineering, and Applied Neuroscience*. CRC Press.

Schramm, F.R. (2025). The Brazilian Bioethics of Protection: Exploring the Old and the New. In: L. Vianna Sobrinho, L. Modolo, M.A. de Santana, G.M. Magalhães Moreno, F.T. Borges, & W.P. dos Santos (Eds.), *Artificial Intelligence and Bioethics: Perspectives*. Routledge.

Sinha, P., Kjelgaard, M.M., Tadin, D. and Held, R. (2017). Autism as a disorder of prediction. *Philosophical Transactions of the Royal Society B: Biological Sciences, 372*(1713), 20160364.

Spinoza, B. (1677/1883). *Ethics, Part I: Concerning God* (R.H.M. Elwes, Trans.). In: R.H.M. Elwes (Ed.), *The Chief Works of Benedict de Spinoza* (Vol. 2). London: G. Bell & Sons. (Original work published 1677.)

Spinoza, B. (1677/1883). *Ethics, Part II: On the Nature and Origin of the Mind* (R.H.M. Elwes, Trans.). In: R.H.M. Elwes (Ed.), *The Chief Works of Benedict de Spinoza* (Vol. 2). London: G. Bell & Sons. (Original work published 1677.)

Spinoza, B. (1677/2025). *Treatise on the Emendation of the Intellect* (R.H.M. Elwes, Trans.). In: R.H.M. Elwes (Ed.), *The Chief Works of Benedict de Spinoza* (Vol. 2). London: G. Bell & Sons. (Original work published 1677.)

Thelwall, M. and Cox, A. (2025). Accuracy of commercial large language model (ChatGPT) to predict the diagnosis for prehospital patients suitable for ambulance transport decisions: Diagnostic accuracy study. *arXiv preprint arXiv:2502.12611*. https://arxiv.org/abs/2502.12611.

Uljarević, M., Evans, J., et al. (2022). Impairments in recognizing all basic facial emotions in autism: A meta-analysis. *Autism, 26*(3), 572–590.

Viana, M.C.M. (2023). *Autismo e intersubjetividade: Um estudo sobre as relações eu-outro-mundo no contexto escolar de um adolescente* (Tese de doutorado, Universidade Federal de Pernambuco). Universidade Federal de Pernambuco, Programa de Pós-Graduação em Psicologia Cognitiva.

Index

About the Editors

Wellington Pinheiro dos Santos is the Head of the Department of Biomedical Engineering at the Federal University of Pernambuco (UFPE) and the Coordinator of the Biomedical Computing Laboratory at UFPE. He holds a Bachelor's degree in Electrical and Electronic Engineering (2001) and a Master's degree in Electrical Engineering (2003) from UFPE, and earned his PhD in Electrical Engineering from the Federal University of Campina Grande in 2009. At UFPE, Dr. dos Santos is actively involved in both undergraduate and graduate programs in Biomedical Engineering. Since 2009, he has also been a member of the Graduate Program in Computer Engineering at the Escola Politécnica de Pernambuco, Universidade de Pernambuco. Additionally, he is a Researcher at the Institute of the Economic-Industrial Complex (ICEIS), where he coordinates the Biomedical Computing and Bioengineering axes. He is a member of the Brazilian Society of Biomedical Engineering (SBEB), the Brazilian Society of Computational Intelligence (SBIC), the Brazilian Society for Health Informatics (SBIS), and the International Federation of Medical and Biological Engineering (IFMBE).

Flávio Secco Fonseca earned his degree in Mechatronics Engineering from the University of Pernambuco in 2017. Currently, he works as a faculty member in the Analysis and Systems Development courses at the Universidade Tiradentes (UNIT). Previously, he was a professor at the Center for Education for Vocational Education (CEPEP). With a focus on Mechatronics and the steel industry, he has experience in Mechanical Engineering. He holds a master's degree in Computer Engineering from the University of Pernambuco (POLI/UPE), conducting research in emotion recognition through voice signals and affective computing. Currently pursuing a Ph.D. at the same institution, he is also part of the Biomedical Computing research group at the Federal University of Pernambuco (UFPE), conducting studies on autism and machine learning. His interests extend to the development of digital games and research in the fields of Educational Technologies, Artificial Intelligence, Health, and Design.

Juliana Carneiro Gomes is a Biomedical Engineer from the Federal University of Pernambuco (UFPE-2016) with a sandwich period under the Science Without Borders program (CAPES) in the United States. During this time, she completed an academic year at Mercer University and worked as a researcher at the Advanced Imaging Algorithms and Instrumentation Laboratory (AIAI Lab) at Johns Hopkins University School of Medicine, gaining experience in Computed Tomography (CT) Image Processing. She holds a Master's degree in Biomedical Engineering from CTG/UFPE (2019), focusing on Electrical Impedance Tomography (EIT) image reconstruction using Artificial Neural Networks. Currently a PhD holder in Computer Engineering at the University of Pernambuco (UPE) and a member of the Biomedical Computing Research Group - UFPE, her research emphasizes applied Neuroscience. Juliana has also served as a substitute professor in the Physics Department at UFPE and was a student representative on the National Commission for Higher Education Assessment (CONAES). Currently, Juliana is a postdoctoral researcher at the Department of Biomedical Engineering (UFPE), a temporary faculty member of the Graduate Program in Biomedical Engineering (UFPE), and a faculty member in the Specialization in Data Science and Digital Health (UFPE).

Maíra Araújo de Santana is a biomedical engineer specializing in artificial intelligence applications in healthcare. She earned her Bachelor's degree in Biomedical Engineering from the Federal University of Pernambuco (UFPE), Brazil, in 2017. During her undergraduate studies, she spent an academic year at the University of Alabama at Birmingham in the United States and worked as a researcher at Duke University's Carl E. Ravin Advanced Imaging Laboratories (RAI Labs), where she developed expertise in medical image processing. Dr. Santana holds a Master's degree in Biomedical Engineering (2020) and a PhD in Computer Engineering (2023) from UFPE. She is currently a postdoctoral researcher and a faculty member in the Specialization in Data Science and Digital Health at the Department of Biomedical Engineering at UFPE. She is a member of the Biomedical Computing Research Group at UFPE, focusing her research on artificial intelligence applied to health. Her work encompasses areas such as pattern recognition for early diagnosis of breast cancer, affective computing, and applied neuroscience.

For Product Safety Concerns and Information please contact our
EU representative GPSR@taylorandfrancis.com Taylor & Francis
Verlag GmbH, Kaufingerstraße 24, 80331 München, Germany